Delmar's Review for the Medical Record Administrator and Technician Certifying Exams

The Health Information Management Series

Delmar Publishers' Online Services
To access Delmar on the World Wide Web, point your browser to:
http://www.delmar.com/delmar.html
To access through Gopher: gopher://gopher.delmar.com
(Delmar Online is part of "thomson.com", an internet site with information on more than 30 publishers of the International Thomson Publishing organization.)
For information on our products and services:
email: info@delmar.com
or call 800-347-7707

Delmar's Review for the Medical Record Administrator and Technician Certifying Exams

The Health Information Management Series

Beth H. Anderson
Kimberly A. Suggs

Shirley Anderson
Series Editor

Delmar Publishers

I(T)P™ An International Thomson Publishing Company

Albany • Bonn • Boston • Cincinnati • Detroit • London • Madrid
Melbourne • Mexico City • New York • Pacific Grove • Paris • San Francisco
Singapore • Tokyo • Toronto • Washington

NOTICE TO THE READER

Publisher does not warrant or guarantee any of the products described herein or perform any independent analysis in connection with any of the product information contained herein. Publisher does not assume, and expressly disclaims, any obligation to obtain and include information other than that provided to it by the manufacturer.

The reader is expressly warned to consider and adopt all safety precautions that might be indicated by the activities described herein and to avoid all potential hazards. By following the instructions contained herein, the reader willingly assumes all risks in connection with such instructions.

The publisher makes no representations or warranties of any kind, including but not limited to, the warranties of fitness for particular purpose or merchantability, nor are any such representations implied with respect to the material set forth herein, and the publisher takes no responsibility with respect to such material. The publisher shall not be liable for any special, consequential or exemplary damages resulting, in whole or in part, from the readers' use of, or reliance upon, this material.

Cover design courtesy: Brucie Rosch

Delmar staff
Publisher: David C. Gordon
Acquisitions Editor: Marion Waldman
Developmental Editor: Jill Rembetski

Project Editor: William Trudell
Production Coordinator: Rich Killar
Marketing Manager: Darryl Caron
Editorial Assistant: Sarah Holle

COPYRIGHT © 1997
By Delmar Publishers
a division of International Thomson Publishing Inc.

The ITP logo is a trademark under license

Printed in the United States of America

For more information, contact:

Delmar Publishers
3 Columbia Circle, Box 15015
Albany, New York 12212-5015

International Thomson Publishing Europe
Berkshire House 168-173
High Holborn
London, WC1V7AA
England

Thomas Nelson Australia
102 Dodds Street
South Melbourne, 3205
Victoria, Australia

Nelson Canada
1120 Birchmount Road
Scarborough, Ontario
Canada M1K 5G4

International Thomson Editores
Campos Eliseos 385, Piso 7
Col Polanco
11560 Mexico D F Mexico

International Thomson Publishing GmbH
Königswinterer Strasse 418
53227 Bonn
Germany

International Thomson Publishing Asia
221 Henderson Road #05-10
Henderson Building
Singapore 0315

International Thomson Publishing - Japan
Hirakawacho Kyowa Building, 3F
2-2-1 Hirakawacho
Chiyoda-ku, 102 Tokyo
Japan

All rights reserved. No part of this work covered by the copyright hereon may be reproduced or used in any form or by any means—graphic, electronic, or mechanical, including photocopying, recording, taping, or information storage and retrieval systems—without written permission of the publisher.

1 2 3 4 5 6 7 8 9 10 XXX 02 01 00 99 98 97 96

Library of Congress Cataloging-in-Publication Data

Anderson, Beth H., 1938–
 Delmar's review for the medical record administrator and technician certifying exams / Beth H. Anderson, Kimberly A. Suggs.
   p   cm. — (The Health information management series)
 Includes bibliographical references.
 ISBN 0-8273-6897-6
 1. Medical records—Management—Examinations, questions, etc.
 I. Suggs, Kimberly A.   II. Title.   III. Series.
 [DNLM:1. Medical Records—examination questions.   2. Forms and Records Control—examination questions.   3. Medical Record Administrators.   4. Certification—United States.   WX 18.2 A545r 1996]
 RA976.A53   1996
 651.5′04261′076—dc20
 DNLM/DLC
 for Library of Congress   95-43921
                                                                                                                                                        CIP

Contents

About the Authors   ix

Acknowledgments   xi

Introduction   xiii

Organization of the Book   xiii
Domains, Tasks, and Competencies   xiv
Content   xv
Levels of Test Items   xvi
Sample Questions   xvi
MRT and MRA Review   xvii
How to Use This Book for Review   xviii

Chapter 1: Test-Taking Strategies   1

Preparing for Review   1
Preparing to Take the Review Tests   1
Tips for Taking the Tests   3
Handling Stress   4

Chapter 2: The Health Record   7

Overview   7
Test Items   9
Answers and Explanations for the Health Record   14
Health Record References for Further Study   16

Chapter 3: Retention and Retrieval   17

Overview   17
Test Items   19
Answers and Explanations for Retention and Retrieval   24
Retention and Retrieval References for Further Study   25

Chapter 4: Health Information Systems   26

Overview   26
Test Items   29
Answers and Explanations for Health Information Systems   35
Health Information Systems References for Further Study   36

Chapter 5: Health-Care Statistics   37

Overview   37
Health-Care Formulas   39
Test Items   41
Answers and Explanations for Health-Care Statistics   46
Health-Care Statistics References for Further Study   48

Chapter 6: Quality of Health Care   49

Overview   49
Test Items   52
Answers and Explanations for Quality of Health Care   58
Quality of Health-Care References for Further Study   60

Chapter 7: Classification Systems   61

Overview   61
Test Items   63
Answers and Explanations for Classification Systems   68
Classification Systems References for Further Study   69

Chapter 8: Coding   70

Overview   70
Test Items   72

Answers and Explanations for Coding   80
Coding References for Further Study   82

Chapter 9: Legal Issues   83

Overview   83
Test Items   85
Answers and Explanations for Legal Issues   91
Legal References for Further Study   93

Chapter 10: Management   94

Overview   94
Test Items   97
Answers and Explanations for Management   104
Management References for Further Study   106

Chapter 11: Human Resource Management   107

Overview   107
Test Items   109
Answers and Explanations for Human Resource Management   115
Human Resource Management References for Further Study   116

Appendices   117

Appendix I: MRA Entry-Level Domains, Tasks, and Competencies   119
Appendix II: MRT Entry-Level Domains, Tasks, and Competencies   126
Appendix III: MRA and MRT Scoring Grids   131

Answer Sheets   135

Practice Exam I Answer Sheets for the MRA and MRT Examinations   137
Practice Exam II Answer Sheets for the MRA and MRT Examinations   159

About the Authors

Beth Anderson, MA, RRA, is currently consulting in the field of health information management and is a quality assessment specialist for the VA External Peer Review Program with the West Virginia Medical Institute, Charleston. She is a former assistant professor and chair of the Department of Health Information Management at the University of Texas Medical Branch, Galveston.

Kimberly Suggs, MS, RRA, is a senior consultant with Ernst and Young in the Dallas office. She is a former instructor and program director at the Department of Health Information Management at the University of Texas Medical Branch, Galveston.

Acknowledgments

We gratefully acknowledge the support of our families and friends who were very tolerant of deadlines and pressures. Valuable assistance was provided by Shirley Anderson, Health Information Management series editor. She gave us many thought-provoking ideas. Jill Rembetski, our developmental editor at Delmar Publishers, was always ready to answer questions and lend encouragement as we struggled with putting this book together. Fellow educators, particularly Barbara Carrington and Rozella Mattingly, were especially supportive of our efforts. We must also acknowledge all those health information management colleagues from who we have learned so much about teaching and, most importantly, how to evaluate students' learning.

Our colleagues who reviewed this book provided very good advice and many excellent suggestions. We would like to acknowledge and thank the following reviewers:

Shirley Anderson, PhD, RRA, Professor, Health Information Management, Saint Louis University, St. Louis, MO

Elizabeth Bowman, MPA, RRA, Associate Professor, Department of Health Information Management, The University of Tennessee, Memphis, Memphis, TN

Melanie Brodnik, PhD, RRA, Director and Assistant Professor, Medical Record Administration, The Ohio State University, Columbus, OH

Debora Butts, MA, RRA, Assistant Professor and Program Director, Health Information Management Program, Texas Southern University, Houston, TX

Eileen Kicken-Dutney, RRA, Program Director, Health Information Technology, Stark Technical College, Canton, OH

Anita Hazelwood, MLS, RRA, Associate Professor, Medical Records Administration Program, The University of Southwestern Louisiana, Lafayette, LA

Margaret Skurka, MS, RRA, CCS, Associate Professor and Director, Health Information Management, Indiana University North West, Gary, IN

Carol Venable, MPH, RRA, Associate Professor, Medical Records Administration Program, The University of Southwestern Louisiana, Lafayette, LA

Introduction

The goal of *Review Book for the MRA and MRT Certification Exams* is to guide you in your preparation for taking the national examinations offered by the American Health Information Management Association (AHIMA). You have completed the education needed to qualify you to write a certifying exam for either a registered record administrator (RRA) or an accredited record technician (ART). The credential will recognize your achievement and allow you to pursue additional opportunities in the rapidly expanding field of health information management.

Organization of the Book

Review Book for the MRA and MRT Certification Exams is organized around the content of the courses that are included in educational programs for health information management. Within these content areas the items will reflect the underlying knowledge required to perform as a health information professional. This review is designed for both the medical record technician (MRT) and the medical record administration (MRA) graduates. The items that apply to MRTs will be at the beginning of each section, with additional items in some chapters for MRAs. The number of items for MRAs and MRTs will be clearly identified so that you will know which questions apply to your review. This book covers the 10 content areas that are included in the national certifying examinations. These areas are identified in the exam results you will receive after taking the national exam.

Domains, Tasks, and Competencies

AHIMA periodically studies the roles and functions that ARTs and RRAs perform during their first year of employment following certification. Such studies identify major areas of responsibilities for the health information management profession. These areas are called domains. The current lists of MRA and MRT domains, tasks, and competencies published in the *1995 Certification Guide* are included as appendices to this book. The roles and functions are under study at the present time and are subject to revision as necessary. The content of this book will include items that test your performance of specific competencies.

This book includes questions that test competencies in all four domains. The number of items from each domain is shown in the accompanying table for both MRAs and MRTs.

	MRA	MRT
Domain 1		
Task 1.1	67	68
Task 1.2	26	26
Task 1.3	33	32
Domain 2		
Task 2.1	24	24
Task 2.2	15	14
Domain 3		
Task 3.1	27	27
Domain 4		
Task 4.1	20	18

In Chapters 2 through 11, the competencies that are tested are identified. This should help you with your review for each chapter.

Content

The 11 chapters of this book are:

√ 1 Test-Taking Strategies
√ 2 The Health Record
√ 3 Retention and Retrieval
   4 Health Information Systems
   5 Health-Care Statistics
   6 Quality of Health Care
   7 Classification Systems
   8 Coding
   9 Legal Issues
  10 Management
  11 Human Resource Management

Chapter 1 gives practical suggestions for preparing for the examination. Strategies for using your time are part of this chapter.

Chapters 2 through 11 test items from a specific course or courses that were part of your educational program. The chapter titles will help you organize the material from the courses you have completed. The courses that you took may have had different titles; however, the same material will have been covered.

Many of the competencies that are listed are applicable to many functional areas within health information management. For example, analyzing a record for utilization review differs from analyzing a record for reimbursement only in the type of information for which you are searching. Other competencies may be omitted from this review because another competency at a higher level was tested. An example of this is competency 1.1.5: Monitor departmental productivity. The competency that is tested is 4.1.2/4.1.1: Determine variation(s) from established objective or standards of performance.

You should review the course notes and exercises by subject to correlate with chapters in this book. This will give you a sound basis for deciding your strengths and weaknesses for content needing further study.

Levels of Test Items

The test items are developed to evaluate different levels of learning. Benjamin S. Bloom (1982) developed such a classification system. AHIMA's national certifying examinations are based on a simplified version which outlines three cognitive levels. The lowest level is the knowledge level. Items at this level evaluate whether you know and understand certain information. Application is the next level tested. Items at this level are used to determine if you can apply information you have learned to situations in the work setting. Problem solving is the highest cognitive level of testing. Items at this level evaluate your ability to synthesize information you have learned, analyze a situation, and use these skills to solve a problem. Examples of test items at these different levels are shown below.

Sample Questions

Knowledge Level

1. *Current Procedural Terminology*, 4th edition (CPT-4), is published and updated by:
   A. AHIMA
   B. American Hospital Association
   C. American Medical Association
   D. JCAHO

Application Level

2. The term used to designate a facility that can be reimbursed by the government for providing services to patients enrolled in the Medicare program is:
   A. Accreditation
   B. Certification
   C. Licensure
   D. Attestation

Problem-Solving Level

3. Transcription equipment costs $80,000 (installed) and requires two people to operate it at an annual cost of $24,000 each, and annual non-labor operating costs are $12,000. Selling transcription services to physicians will result in $165,000 revenue the first year. The expected gross income (loss) for the first year is
   A. ($59,000)
   B. ($25,000)
   C. $25,000
   D. $59,000

Correct Answers and Sources/Explanation for Sample Questions

1. C *Source:* Huffman (1994), pages 329–331.
2. B *Source:* Huffman (1994), pages 10–12.
3. C $165,000 − [$80,000 + ($24,000 × 2) + $12,000]

MRT and MRA Review

All test items are appropriate for those who are preparing for the MRA certification exam. Items that apply to the examination for MRTs will be listed first and the number of items clearly identified at the beginning of each set of questions. In the Appendix, two copies of answer sheets are provided to be used when preparing for the RRA certifying exam and two copies are provided to be used when preparing for the ART certifying exam. Remove these from the book and discard the set that does not apply to the exam for which you are preparing. You can work through the review book and answer the items using one set of the answer sheets. You can use the second set of answer sheets to take the tests a second time after you have done further review.

The answers are provided following each series of test items in each content area. The level of the item (knowledge, application, or problem solving) will also be shown as will the explanation or source for the answer. The competencies from the domains and tasks will also be identified for each question. When only one competency is listed, it is the same for both MRA and MRT. If the competencies are different, the MRA competency will be listed first, followed by the MRT competency.

The chapters also include references for further study. You may only have a few of these in your collection. By using other reference materials you can broaden your knowledge in any of these areas.

How to Use This Book for Review

Before you begin working through the problems in this book you should gather the texts and other materials from your courses. You should organize these materials by courses. This will make your review easier and will also let you refer to them as necessary after you have completed each section. Also have a copy of *Health Information Management*, 10th edition (Huffman, 1994), on hand for reference. As you begin each chapter, first review the relevant information from your notes before answering the questions. Be sure to review Chapter 1 before you begin to answer any test items.

Use the answer sheets provided to record your answers. The questions are all multiple choice and you will choose the one best answer for each item. Mark either A, B, C, or D for each question number. Be sure to show any problem solving you did, either beside the question or on a separate sheet of paper. This will help you retrace your steps and let you determine whether you made a careless error in math or reading. If you make many of these kinds of errors, you will want to refer to Chapter 1 again, which reviews test-taking strategies. You will also want to note if you had to guess at the answer by placing a question mark or other symbol beside the question. Guessing is an important clue that you may need more information about this topic.

After you answer each series of questions, check your choices against the answers and explanations provided at the end of the chapter. A scoring grid is provided with the answer sheets so that you can determine your score for each chapter and your overall score. You will want to do further review in those areas where you record the lowest scores. References for study are provided after each series of test items.

These questions are not from the national examination. They are only examples of the types of questions that the examination contains. The national exam will contain different questions that test these areas of knowledge.

Remember that you have been successful this far in pursuing your career goals. Your instructors have provided many opportunities for you to analyze and synthesize information and to develop problem-solving skills. Use the skills you have developed in your education. This book can help you determine your strengths and weaknesses so that you can use your time wisely as you prepare for the examination.

References

Bloom, B. S. 1982. Reprint ed. *Taxonomy of educational objectives.* London: Longman.

Huffman, E. K. (1994). *Health information management* (10th ed.). Berwyn, IL: Physician's Record Company.

Chapter 1

Test-Taking Strategies

Preparing for Review

Using this book for review will help you organize your studies and use your time wisely. A suggested time line for conducting your review is shown in Table 1-1. This schedule is designed for a person who is working and will be studying 2 to 4 hours for 6 days each week. If you are not working you may choose to complete more than this schedule outlines for each week. The important thing is to pace your review so that you feel more comfortable when you take the exam.

However you schedule your review, be sure that you study only for 45 or 50 minutes and then take a break. This will allow you to concentrate on what you are studying. If possible, study in a room where your materials can be organized and you can be alone without distractions such as a phone or television. You will want to use a timer and give yourself breaks as appropriate.

Preparing to Take the Review Tests

Before you begin answering the questions in each section make sure you have pencils and a calculator ready. At the certifying exam you are told to have #2 pencils for marking the score sheets. It is a good idea to take all the review tests the same way.

The AHIMA certification exam for registered record administrators is normally 4.5 hours in length and has 250 questions. The AHIMA certification exam for accredited record technicians is 4.25 hours in length and has

Table 1-1. Suggested Time Line for Review

Time	Activity
Week 1	Read Preface and Chapter 1 Organize material, develop personal time line
Week 2	Read Overview for Chapters 2 and 3 Review material for Chapters 2 and 3 Complete Chapters 2 and 3
Week 3	Read Overview for Chapters 4 and 5 Review material for Chapters 4 and 5 Complete Chapters 4 and 5
Week 4	Read Overview for Chapters 6 and 7 Review material for Chapters 6 and 7 Complete Chapters 6 and 7
Week 5	Read Overview for Chapter 8 Review material for Chapter 8 Complete Chapter 8
Week 6	Read Overview for Chapters 9 and 10 Review material for Chapters 9 and 10 Complete Chapters 9 and 10
Week 7	Read Overview for Chapter 11 Review material for Chapter 11 Complete Chapter 11
Week 8	Review Scores Determine where further study is needed Perform further study/review
Week 9	Use new set of answer sheets to complete Chapters 2 through 11
Week 10	Relax and prepare yourself mentally and physically for examination

200 questions. In this book you will be given a time limit for each section that is in proportion to the time allowed for each exam. This will allow you to practice answering questions with a time limit similar to that of the national examination.

Tips for Taking the Tests

1. Use #2 pencils for all practice exams. This will prepare you for AHIMA MRA/MRT examinations.
2. Do not make any marks on the answer sheet except inside the circle of the answer you have chosen.
3. You can write in the examination booklet during AHIMA certifying examinations. Prepare yourself for doing this by writing in the review book. Do computations, jot notes to yourself, and place question marks when you are unsure. As time permits, review unsure items marked with a question mark.
4. Read each question carefully. It can be helpful to use your pencil as a guide to help control your anxiety and to keep you from skipping words.
5. Do not read more into a question than is stated. If you have a habit of doing this, use the practice questions to try to eliminate this behavior.
6. Cover the answer choices and answer the question before looking at the options. This will reduce the distraction of the wrong answers.
7. Use your time effectively. You will have less than a minute for each item. If you are a slow test taker you will want to monitor your progress as you work through this review book. Then, when you take the national examination, you can feel more confident that you will have enough time for the test. You might help yourself stay within the time frame by writing target times in the booklet as you begin the exam. For instance, if the exam starts at 9:00 A.M. you can write 9:45 beside item number 50 in the exam booklet. When you get to this question you can check your progress and adjust as necessary.
8. All examination items in this review book and on AHIMA's certifying examination are multiple choice with four possible answers. Choose the one **best** answer.
9. The stem of the item is the part that tells you what question you should answer. Select one of the four possible responses.

Example

To illustrate percentage of total patients discharged for each source of payment, the recommended chart would be:

A. Box plot (Tukey)
B. Bar chart
C. Line chart
D. Pie chart

The stem describes an example of presenting data and the choices list different charts that are used in analyzing data. The correct response is D. The other three choices are called distractors. The distractor should appear to be plausible choices to someone who does not know the answer. If you know that box plots are used to show the distribution of a sample, you can eliminate answer A. By eliminating one answer your chance of correctly answering the question rises from one out of four (or 25%) to one out of three (33%).

10. When you find an item that you cannot answer quickly, put a question mark beside that question and move on. Time is limited and you do not want to waste time on an item that has you baffled. You can return to this item later if you have time.

11. When the question involves a scenario, read the questions first before reading the scenario. This will focus your reading in the right direction.

12. Answer all questions. It is better to guess than to leave an item unanswered. An unanswered item will be wrong. A guess has a 25% chance of being correct.

13. Do not change answers. Except for items that you have marked with a question mark, it is generally better to leave your initial choice.

Handling Stress

Take Care of Your Body

Eat three balanced meals each day during the week prior to the examination. Carbohydrates play an important part in our diet. Digestion breaks down carbohydrates into glucose, the major source of fuel for muscles and the only source of energy for the brain. Choose unrefined carbohydrates, such as whole grains and brown rice. Include vegetables, beans, and corn, which are also carbohydrates.

Be sure to eat a good breakfast the day of the exam. Avoid excess liquids on exam day to minimize the need for trips to the bathroom. Get plenty of sleep the week prior to the examination, particularly the three nights immediately preceding the test.

Wear comfortable clothes and shoes to the examination. Carry a light wrap or sweater in case the examination room is chilly. This way you will decrease the chance that you will be distracted by discomfort. If you wear contacts or glasses, be sure to carry an extra pair of glasses to the examination.

Calm Your Mind

Proper preparation reduces anxiety. The program where you completed your education has covered the material that you need for successful completion of the certifying examination. By completing this book you will review all relevant material. Feel sure that you have the knowledge necessary to pass this exam. A positive attitude will do much to relieve unnecessary anxiety.

Rehearse the route to the examination site. It is best to do this at the same time of day on the Saturday before the exam. Include parking your car and locating the registration area in the rehearsal and in time estimates. Add another 30 minutes to the rehearsal time for unexpected delays. This will keep your anxiety level lower and will also allow you time to locate the bathroom before the exam. If you must travel to the examination site, make your rehearsal run the evening prior to the exam.

Be sure that your admission ticket, a picture ID, extra glasses, battery-operated calculator with extra batteries, ICD-9-CM and CPT-4 coding books, several pencils, and a good eraser are packed in a briefcase, ready to carry to the examination.

Practice relaxation techniques and exercises. Many good books and tapes are available. Begin these as you work through this review book. Focus on methods you can use at the testing site—remember you cannot have a tape recorder there.

Use your favorite relaxation method anytime during the review when you feel your anxiety level rising. That way the exercise will be very familiar to you and you can use it the day of the national certifying exam. Before the examination begins, you can help yourself relax. Then, throughout the examination when your anxiety level begins to rise, you can use the exercise to help calm yourself.

Because of your preparation for this important examination you will be much more relaxed and confident. You deserve to pass the exam and we believe you will!

Chapter 2

The Health Record

Overview

The items in this chapter test your knowledge of the contents of the health record and requirements for those contents. How the record is organized, what reports are commonly found in the record, and what these reports should contain are all knowledge that you will need in order to analyze the record. Analysis of records requires that you apply the knowledge you gained in human anatomy, medical terminology, and pathophysiology.

The particular competencies that are tested in this chapter are listed below, both for MRAs and MRTs.

MRA Competencies

1.1.9   Collect data on the quality of documentation in the medical record (i.e., timeliness, completeness, accuracy).
1.1.26 Perform concurrent medical record review.
1.2.2   Verify timeliness, completeness, accuracy, and appropriateness of data sources (patient care, management, billing reports, or databases).
1.2.4   Check data for internal consistency.
1.2.5   Perform edit checks to monitor data accuracy.
1.3.4   Analyze patient care/institutional data in relation to regulatory and accreditation standards.
1.3.6   Analyze physician performance data/profiles in relation to medical staff, institutional, or regulatory or accreditation standards.

MRT Competencies

1.1.9   Collect data on the quality of documentation in the medical record (i.e., timeliness, completeness, accuracy).
1.1.28 Perform concurrent medical record review.
1.2.2   Verify timeliness, completeness, accuracy, and appropriateness of data sources (patient care, management, billing reports, or databases).
1.2.4   Check data for internal consistency.
1.2.5   Perform edit checks to monitor data accuracy.
1.3.3   Analyze patient care/institutional data in relation to regulatory and accreditation standards.

Before you answer the questions, review your course material including all handouts, exercises, quizzes, and texts. Also review chapters 2 through 6 in *Health Information Management,* 10th edition (Huffman, 1994).

Use one of the answer sheets provided for Chapter 2 to record your answers. Choose the one best answer for each item. Mark either A, B, C, or D for each question number.

Be sure to show any problem solving you did, either beside the question in the review book or on a separate sheet of paper. This will help you retrace your steps and let you determine whether you made a careless error in math or reading. If you make many of these kinds of errors, you will want to refer to Chapter 1 again, which reviews test-taking strategies. You will also want to note if you had to guess at the answer by placing a question mark or other symbol beside the question. Guessing is an important clue that you may need more information about this topic.

After you answer the questions, check your choices against the answers and explanations provided at the end of the chapter. Use the number of questions that you answered correctly to calculate your score using the grid on the answer sheet. Do not waste time fretting over your score at this point in the review. This would be a good time to indicate those materials you would like to review further before the national exam.

Place the score for this chapter on the separate grid that is provided. The grid will allow you to determine your overall score when you have completed all the tests. You will want to do further review in those areas where you record the lowest scores. References for further study are provided at the end of each chapter.

Test Items

Health Record Questions

Number of Items: 20
MRA Time Allowed: 18 minutes
MRT Time Allowed: 19 minutes

Start

1. According to JCAHO, a complete history and physical would NOT be required in which of the following cases:
   A. Patient is readmitted after being discharged 7 days ago with a diagnosis of angina pectoris. The provisional diagnosis for the readmission is cerebrovascular accident.
   B. Patient is admitted for uncomplicated OB delivery after only one prenatal visit 7 months ago.
   C. Complete work-up for elective hysterectomy (including lab and x-rays) was performed 5 days ago in the physician's office. A copy of the history and physical completed at that time were sent to the hospital.
   D. Left cataract surgery was performed 6 weeks ago and the patient is now present for right cataract surgery.

2. A regulatory agency requires that a record contain a Review of Systems. Within the medical record, this inventory by systems would be located in the:
   A. Discharge summary
   B. Doctor's orders
   C. History
   D. Physical examination

3. A statement likely to be found in the physical examination report is:
   A. "Admission white blood count was 14,000."
   B. "Moist rales were heard in both lung bases."
   C. "Cholecystectomy was done 3 years ago."
   D. "The patient was admitted because of pain in the right upper quadrant."

4. You have been asked to provide a patient's respiratory rates for the first, second, and fifth days in the hospital. The quickest way to locate this information would be to review the:
   A. Graphic record (TPR)
   B. Nurses' notes
   C. Physician's progress notes for the first, second, and fifth days
   D. Nursing care plan

5. A final progress note may substitute for a discharge summary for a patient:
   A. Admitted for overnight observation following a trauma to the head
   B. Admitted for a normal obstetric labor and delivery
   C. Admitted for colonoscopy who dies 36 hours after admission
   D. Admitted for gastroplasty whose surgery is canceled because of an episode of hyperthermia following induction of anesthesia

6. JCAHO requires physicians to authenticate (or sign) telephone orders, which are known to be hazardous to the patient. The time frame for such authentication is:
   A. Within 24 hours
   B. Within 48 hours
   C. Within 72 hours
   D. That specified in the medical staff rules and regulations

7. An APGAR score will most probably be found in the medical record of a:
   A. Cardiac patient
   B. Chronic obstructive lung disease patient
   C. Newborn patient
   D. Renal disease patient

8. The listing of several different diagnoses from which the patient may be suffering is the:
   A. Differential diagnosis
   B. Impression
   C. Preoperative diagnosis
   D. Tentative diagnosis

9. Laboratory tests are very important diagnostic tools. When such tests are necessary they are ordered by the:
   A. Medical technologist
   B. Nursing supervisor
   C. Physician
   D. Pathologist

10. To correct an error in the medical record the individual who made the error should:
    A. Draw a line through the error, add a note explaining the error, and date and initial the correction
    B. Totally mark through the error, correct it, and have the attending physician sign the correction
    C. Rewrite or type the page again where the error was located and then get the page resigned
    D. Use correction fluid to cover the error and add the correct information, leaving the date and signature for the original entry

11. The integrated medical record is identified by its:
    A. Arrangement according to hospital departments
    B. Strict chronological order
    C. Association of treatment with specific problems
    D. Inclusion of insurance and business record

12. A medical staff has been concerned with the quality of progress notes in the patient's records and recommends institution of SOAP progress notes. In a SOAP progress note, the statement "complaining of severe headaches" would be in this part of the note:
    A. Subjective
    B. Objective
    C. Assessment
    D. Plan

13. The main advantage of having a medical record report dictated and transcribed is that it:
    A. Improves its legibility
    B. Increases its accuracy
    C. Increases its timeliness
    D. Reduces its cost to the organization

14. A hospital averages 250 discharges during the 2-week period allowed for completion of medical records. When data are compiled for the most recent 2-week period, there are 195 incomplete records and 75 delinquent records. The delinquent rate for this period is:
    A. 0.30%
    B. 0.78%
    C. 30.00%
    D. 78.00%

15. One of the basic components of quantitative analysis is:
    A. Consistency of entries by all health-care providers
    B. Presence of all necessary reports
    C. Justification for the patient's hospital course
    D. Occurrence of a potentially compensable event

16. The interdisciplinary comprehensive care plan is normally part of:
    A. Home health records
    B. Hospice records
    C. Long-term-care records
    D. Mental health records

17. As HIM manager you are developing a quantitative analysis procedure for a hospice unit that your organization is planning to open next month. Medicare regulations require that a hospice record must at least include:
    A. Assessment once a week
    B. Home health treatment plan
    C. Review of documentation every 7 days
    D. Summary of all inpatient services when provided

18. Medical records that include the emotional and behavioral, legal, vocational, and recreational assessments are found in a:
    A. Home health facility
    B. Hospice
    C. Long-term-care facility
    D. Mental health facility

19. While performing qualitative analysis on a patient's medical record you see a positive laboratory report identifying the organism as *Treponema pallidum*. You would expect to see a diagnosis of:
    A. Brucellosis
    B. Gas gangrene
    C. Gonorrhea
    D. Syphilis

20. JCAHO standards for the management of information specify that operative reports should be written or dictated for the medical record:
    A. During recovery room status
    B. Immediately after surgery
    C. Within 24 hours of surgery
    D. Within 15 days of surgery

Stop

Answers and Explanations for the Health Record

1. **C** *Level:* Application   *Competency:* 1.3.4/1.3.3
   Source: Huffman (1994), page 64.

2. **C** *Level:* Knowledge   *Competency:* 1.3.4/1.3.3
   Source: Huffman (1994), page 60.

3. **B** *Level:* Application   *Competency:* 1.1.26/1.1.28
   Rationale: A description of breath sounds is given in section on lungs in the physical examination.
   Source: Huffman (1994), page 64.

4. **A** *Level:* Application   *Competency:* 1.1.26/1.1.28
   Source: Huffman (1994), pages 82–83.

5. **B** *Level:* Application   *Competency:* 1.3.4/1.3.3
   Rationale: The patients described in answers A, C, and D are not uncomplicated cases.
   Source: Huffman (1994), page 79.

6. **D** *Level:* Knowledge   *Competency:* 1.3.4/1.3.3
   Source: Huffman (1994), page 65.

7. **C** *Level:* Application   *Competency:* 1.1.26/1.1.28
   Source: Huffman (1994), page 98.

8. **A** *Level:* Knowledge   *Competency:* 1.1.26/1.1.28
   Source: Huffman (1994), page 63.

9. **C** *Level:* Knowledge   *Competency:* 1.2.2
   Source: Huffman (1994), page 84.

10. **A** *Level:* Knowledge   *Competency:* 1.2.5
    Source: Huffman (1994), pages 108, 230.

11. **B** *Level:* Knowledge   *Competency:* 1.1.26/1.1.28
    Source: Huffman (1994), page 104.

12. **A** *Level:* Application *Competency:* 1.2.2
    Rationale: This is obviously a quote from the patient and, as such, is subjective information.
    Source: Huffman (1994), page 104.

13. **A** *Level:* Knowledge *Competency:* 1.1.9
    Source: Huffman (1994), page 108.

14. **C** *Level:* Application *Competency:* 1.3.6/1.3.3
    Rationale: 75/250 = 0.30 X 100 (to determine percent delinquent). The percent delinquent is merely the number of delinquent records compared to the total number of discharges for the period.
    Source: Huffman (1994), page 239.

15. **B** *Level:* Knowledge *Competency:* 1.2.2
    Source: Huffman (1994), page 228.

16. **C** *Level:* Knowledge *Competency:* 1.1.26/1.1.28
    Source: Huffman (1994), page 156.

17. **D** *Level:* Knowledge *Competency:* 1.3.4/1.3.3
    Source: Huffman (1994), page 181.

18. **D** *Level:* Knowledge *Competency:* 1.1.26/1.1.28
    Source: Huffman (1994), pages 202–203.

19. **D** *Level:* Application *Competency:* 1.2.4
    Rationale: Treponema pallidum is a gram-negative organism that is the causative agent for syphilis in humans.
    Source: Dorland's Illustrated Medical Dictionary.

20. **C** *Level:* Knowledge *Competency:* 1.3.4/1.3.3
    Source: 1995 Accreditation Manual for Hospitals.

Health Record References for Further Study

Dorland's illustrated medical dictionary, (28th ed.). (1994). Philadelphia: W. B. Saunders.

Glondys, B. (1993). *Documentation requirements for the acute care patient record.* Chicago: American Health Information Management Association.

Huffman, E. K. (1994). *Health information management* (10th ed.). Berwyn, IL: Physicians' Record Company.

Joint Commission on Accreditation of Healthcare Organizations (1994). *1995 Accreditation manual for hospitals. Volume 1: Standards.* Oakbrook, IL: Joint Commission on Accreditation of Healthcare Organizations.

Manano, J. (Ed.). (1993). *Health information management: A comprehensive guide to current regulations and management practices.* Los Angeles: Practice Management Information Corporation.

Skurka, M. (1994). *Health information management in hospitals.* Chicago, IL: American Hospital Association.

Chapter 3

Retention and Retrieval

Overview

This chapter deals with the filing, storage, and retrieval of patients' records, as well as tracking the location of records, including all the guidelines for alphabetic, terminal digit, and straight numeric filing methods. You will also want to review how to determine storage needs for card files, patient records, and microfilm. The maintenance of indexes and registers is also included in this chapter.

The particular competencies that are tested in this chapter are listed below, both for MRAs and MRTs.

MRA Competencies

1.1.21 Abstract information from patient records (concurrently or retrospectively) for disease, procedure, physician, or other indices.
1.1.22 Abstract information from patient records (concurrently or retrospectively) for compilation of registries.
2.1.4 Develop or revise departmental procedures.
2.2.8 Determine space requirements for current or new systems.
3.1.6 Implement new or revised information, service, or operational systems.

Chapter 3

MRT Competencies

1.1.22 Abstract information from patient records (concurrently or retrospectively) for disease, procedure, physician, or other indices.
1.1.23 Abstract information from patient records (concurrently or retrospectively) for compilation of registries.
2.1.3 Develop or revise departmental procedures.
2.2.3 Determine space requirements for current or new systems.
3.1.6 Implement new or revised information, service, or operational systems.

Before you answer the questions, review your course material including all handouts, exercises, quizzes, and texts. Also review chapters 8 and 10 in *Health Information Management*, 10th edition (Huffman, 1994). Answering the questions in this chapter will help the reader review knowledge and skills about retention and retrieval of health records.

Use one of the answer sheets provided for Chapter 3 to record your answers. Choose the one best answer for each item. Mark either A, B, C, or D for each question number.

Again, be sure to show any problem solving you did, either beside the question in the review book or on a separate sheet of paper. This will help you retrace your steps and let you determine whether you made a careless error in math or reading. If you continue to make many of these kinds of errors, refer to Chapter 1 again, which reviews test-taking strategies. Also note if you had to guess at the answer by placing a question mark or other symbol beside the question. Guessing is an important clue that you may need more information about this topic.

After you answer the questions, check your choices against the answers and explanations provided at the end of the chapter. Use the number of questions that you answered correctly to calculate your score using the grid on the answer sheet. Again mark those references that you would like to review further before the national exam.

Place the score for this chapter on the separate grid that is provided. The grid will allow you to determine your overall score when you have completed all the tests. You will want to do further review in those areas where you record the lowest scores. References for study are provided at the end of the chapter.

Test Items

Retention and Retrieval Questions

Number of Items: 20
MRA Time Allowed: 18 minutes
MRT Time Allowed: 19 minutes

Start

1. A patient is admitted in 1992 and receives number 16-43-01. She is readmitted in 1993 and receives number 18-41-12. The record with the number 16-43-01 is brought forward to 18-41-12. This is an example of:
   A. Family numbering and filing
   B. Serial numbering and filing
   C. Serial unit numbering and filing
   D. Unit numbering and filing

2. When filing in terminal digit order, the number of the folders immediately before and behind the folder numbered 24-21-83 will be:
   A. 24-21-82 and 24-21-84
   B. 24-11-83 and 24-31-83
   C. 23-21-83 and 25-21-83
   D. 24-20-83 and 24-22-83

3. In a facility with a unit numbering system and a terminal digit filing system, Mrs. Dahlwhite, a new patient, was just issued number 24-53-68. The next number issued to a new patient will be:
   A. 25-53-68
   B. 25-53-69
   C. 24-54-68
   D. 24-53-69

4. When planning to make guides for every secondary number in a terminal digit file, the lowest secondary number for the 99 primary section will be:
   A. 00
   B. 01
   C. 10
   D. 99

5. The filing and numbering system that results in records of different admissions for the same patient being filed in more than one location is:
   A. Serial numbering and filing
   B. Serial terminal digit numbering and filing
   C. Serial unit numbering and filing
   D. Unit numbering and filing

6. The following is the sequence of records in a record file.

   11-43-97
   11-43-98
   11-43-99
   11-44-00
   11-44-01

   This is an example of:
   A. Middle digit filing
   B. Reverse numeric filing
   C. Straight numeric filing
   D. Terminal digit filing

7. A filing supervisor has had an increasing problem with misfiled records. One of the best methods for reducing the number of misfiled records is:
   A. Installing movable shelving
   B. Converting to color-coded file folders
   C. Changing the numbering system
   D. Hiring someone to continually check the files

8. The complete medical record of a patient in a serial unit system is obtained by:
   A. Looking under each number assigned to the patient
   B. Looking under the most recently assigned number
   C. Looking under the number assigned on the first admission
   D. None of the above

9. Purging inactive records from the file is easiest when using:
   A. Middle digit filing
   B. Serial numbering and filing
   C. Terminal digit filing
   D. Unit numbering and filing

10. In a small department that is very short of available space for filing and storage of patient records it is best to use:
    A. Six-drawer lateral files
    B. Five-drawer vertical file cabinets
    C. Fixed open shelving
    D. Movable open shelving

11. In master patient index Dr. James M. Dominque would be filed as:
    A. Dominque, James M. (Dr.)
    B. Dominque, J. James (Dr.)
    C. James M. Dominque (Dr.)
    D. Dr. James M. Dominque

12. A small hospital has approximately 50,000 inpatient admissions each year, an emergency department, a day surgery service, but no outpatient clinics. This facility does not have a sophisticated computer system. Considering both the cost and the need for strict record control, the best method for chart tracking in this situation would be:
    A. A log book where a list of records taken from the department is kept
    B. A policy that does not allow records to be removed from the filing area
    C. A charge-out system with an outguide replacing any record removed
    D. An automated record tracking system

13. A large urban hospital has four satellite outpatient clinics. The active and inactive records for these outpatient clinics are maintained at each of the four satellite sites. Policies and procedures for all sites are the same as those used in the hospital setting. This form of organization is referred to as:
    A. Centralized
    B. Controlled-decentralized
    C. Decentralized
    D. Satellite

14. Permanent retention of copies of daily admission lists is a satisfactory substitute for the:
   A. Number index
   B. Daily patient census
   C. Patient admission register
   D. Master patient index

15. In a Health Information Management (HIM) department there are 85,000 records. It is the department standard to have 100 records between guides for a terminal digit system. To meet this standard you will need:
   A. 85 guides
   B. 425 guides
   C. 850 guides
   D. 8500 guides

16. The following names are to be filed alphabetically.

   H. Smith
   Frances Smithe
   Joseph S. Smithe
   Joseph Smith

   The name that should be filed third is:
   A. H. Smith
   B. Frances Smithe
   C. Joseph S. Smithe
   D. Joseph Smith

17. In a cancer registry, the specific treatment received by a patient would be found in the:
   A. Master index file
   B. Accession register
   C. Case files
   D. Follow-up file

18. You have received a request from a physician for a list of all of the patients she has treated at your facility during the past year. To identify those patients you would use the:
   A. Disease and operation index
   B. Physician's index
   C. Master patient index
   D. Patient admission register

19. A nursing home is remodeling the filing area for patient records. To store the records currently being maintained, 1320 inches are required. An additional 495 inches must be added to allow for expansion during the next 5 years. The shelving units that are being purchased will hold 165 linear inches of records. The number of shelving units that should be purchased to house the present records plus those expected during the next 5 years is:
    A. 3
    B. 5
    C. 8
    D. 11

20. HIM department microfilmed 5000 inactive records that on average contained 72 pages and were ½ inch thick. The method used was microfiche. Each microfiche holds 98 images filmed at a reduction ratio of 24×. A total of 100 microfiche can be filed in 1 inch. The space required to file these microfiche is approximately:
    A. 25 inches
    B. 50 inches
    C. 250 inches
    D. 500 inches

Stop

24 Chapter 3

Answers and Explanations for Retention and Retrieval

1. **C** *Level:* Application *Competency:* 2.1.4/2.1.3
   Source: Huffman (1994), page 277.

2. **C** *Level:* Application *Competency:* 2.1.4/2.1.3
   Source: Huffman (1994), pages 284–287.

3. **D** *Level:* Application *Competency:* 2.1.4/2.1.3
   Source: Huffman (1994), page 277.

4. **A** *Level:* Application *Competency:* 2.1.4/2.1.3
   Source: Huffman (1994), page 285.

5. **A** *Level:* Application *Competency:* 2.1.4/2.1.3
   Source: Huffman (1994), pages 276–277.

6. **C** *Level:* Application *Competency:* 2.1.4/2.1.3
   Source: Huffman (1994), page 284.

7. **B** *Level:* Knowledge *Competency:* 3.1.6
   Source: Huffman (1994), page 391.

8. **B** *Level:* Application *Competency:* 2.1.4/2.1.3
   Source: Huffman (1994), page 277.

9. **B** *Level:* Application *Competency:* 2.1.4/2.1.3
   Source: Huffman (1994), page 282.

10. **D** *Level:* Application *Competency:* 2.2.8/2.2.3
    Source: Huffman (1994), page 290.

11. **A** *Level:* Application *Competency:* 2.1.4/2.1.3
    Source: Huffman (1994), pages 370–371.

12. **C** *Level:* Application *Competency:* 2.1.4/2.1.3
    Rationale: A charge-out system using outguides in the file would also include some sort of centralized chart tracking (which might be a log book or carbon copies of requests). This method would be the most economical if computer support is not available. A log book by itself is not a complete charge tracking system.
    Source: Huffman (1994), pages 296–300.

13. **B** *Level:* Application   *Competency:* 2.1.4/2.1.3
    Source: Huffman (1994), pages 294–296.

14. **C** *Level:* Application   *Competency:* 2.1.4/2.1.3
    Source: Huffman (1994), pages 383–384.

15. **C** *Level:* Application   *Competency:* 2.1.4/2.1.3
    Rationale: 85,000/100 = 850 guides
    Source: Huffman (1994), page 291.

16. **B** *Level:* Application   *Competency:* 2.1.4/2.1.3
    Source: Huffman (1994), pages 370–381.

17. **C** *Level:* Application   *Competency:* 1.1.22/1.1.23
    Source: Huffman (1994), pages 385–389.

18. **B** *Level:* Application   *Competency:* 1.1.21/1.1.22
    Source: Huffman (1994), pages 381–383.

19. **D** *Level:* Problem Solving   *Competency:* 2.2.8/2.2.3
    Rationale: (1320 + 495)/165 = 11 shelving units needed
    Source: Huffman (1994), pages 289–290.

20. **B** *Level:* Problem solving   *Competency:* 2.2.8/2.2.3
    Rationale: One microfiche will hold an average record of 72 pages; therefore, 5000 records will require 5000 microfiche. 5000/100 = 50 inches required.
    Source: Huffman (1994), pages 313–314.

Retention and Retrieval References for Further Study

Huffman, E. K. (1994). *Health information management* (10th ed.). Berwyn, IL: Physicians' Record Company.

Kallaus, N. F. & Keeling, B. L. (1991). *Administrative office management* (10th ed.). Cincinnati, OH: South-Western Publishing Co.

Chapter 4

Health Information Systems

Overview

The focus of this chapter is on the development and use of computer systems to collect health data. Included are aspects of systems analysis, including the request for proposal (RFP), as well as knowledge about hardware and software.

Data definitions are important when talking about health information systems. Software that is appropriate to manipulate, analyze, and display data is also important when discussing health information systems. What software to use in different situations is one of the critical elements included in this chapter.

The particular competencies that are tested in this chapter are listed below, both for MRAs and MRTs.

MRA Competencies

1.1.20 Abstract information from patient records (concurrently or retrospectively) for reimbursement.
1.2.5   Perform edit checks to monitor data accuracy.
1.3.6   Analyze physician performance data/profiles in relation to medical staff, institutional, or regulatory or accreditation standards.
2.1.8   Develop transition plans for implementation of new or revised systems.
2.1.16 Develop goals and objectives for computerized information systems (i.e., department or other facility systems).
2.2.6   Determine personnel needs for staffing current or new systems.

2.2.7 Determine equipment or supply needs for current or new systems.
2.2.8 Determine space requirements for current or new systems.
3.1.6 Implement new or revised information, service, or operational systems.
3.1.7 Monitor adherence to budget (i.e., determine budget variance, etc.).
3.1.9 Monitor policy or procedure compliance.
4.1.1 Monitor system outcomes (i.e., benefits, costs, etc.).
4.1.3 Recommend changes or improvement(s) in systems.

MRT Competencies

1.1.21 Abstract information from patient records (concurrently or retrospectively) for reimbursement.
1.2.5   Perform edit checks to monitor data accuracy.
1.3.6   Analyze physician performance data/profiles in relation to medical staff, institutional, or regulatory or accreditation standards.
2.1.5   Develop transition plans for implementation of new or revised systems.
2.1.6   Develop goals and objectives for computerized information systems (i.e., department or other facility systems).
2.2.1   Determine personnel needs for staffing current or new systems.
2.2.2   Determine equipment or supply needs for current or new systems.
2.2.3   Determine space requirements for current or new systems.
3.1.6   Implement new or revised information, service, or operational systems.
3.1.7   Monitor adherence to budget (i.e., determine budget variance, etc.).
3.1.9   Monitor policy or procedure compliance.
4.1.2   Recommend changes or improvement(s) in systems.

Before you answer the questions, review your course material including all handouts, exercises, quizzes, and texts. Also review chapters 13 and 14 in *Health Information Management,* 10th edition (Huffman, 1994). Answering the questions in this chapter will help the reader review knowledge and skills about health information systems.

Use one of the answer sheets provided for Chapter 4 to record your answers. Choose the one best answer for each item. Mark either A, B, C, or D for each question number.

Again, be sure to show any problem solving you did, either beside the question in the review book or on a separate sheet of paper. This will help you retrace your steps and let you determine whether you made a careless error in math or reading. If you continue to make many of these kinds of errors, refer to Chapter 1 again, which reviews test-taking strategies. Also note if you had to guess at the answer by placing a question mark or other symbol beside the question. Guessing is an important clue that you may need more information about this topic.

After you answer the questions, check your choices against the answers and explanations provided. Use the number of questions that you answered correctly to calculate your score using the grid on the answer sheet. Again indicate those materials that you would like to review further before the national exam.

Place the score for this chapter on the separate grid that is provided. The grid will allow you to determine your overall score when you have completed all the tests. You will want to do further review in those areas where you record the lowest scores. References for study are provided at the end of the chapter.

Test Items

Health Information Systems Questions

Number of Items: 17 MRA/14 MRT (Omit last 3 questions)
MRA Time Allowed: 16 minutes
MRT Time Allowed: 13 minutes

Start

1. A manager has the capability of printing ad hoc reports from the automated abstracting system. A request from the vice president for planning asks for the following information: the number of outpatients seen in the last 6 months from each of three zip codes, the code number of the attending physician, and the patient's last name. File definitions for this database are given below:

Field Name	Values	Description
Zip Code	All valid zip codes	Nine digits
Type of Patient	1 2	Inpatient Outpatient
Physician	100–999	Three digits (Ex: 123)
Date of Treatment	All valid dates	xx/xx/xxxx
Patient Name		15 alpha characters

In responding to this request, values must be specified for the following fields:

A. Type of patient, physician code number, and date of treatment
B. Date of treatment, zip code, and patient's name
C. Zip code, date of treatment, and type of patient
D. Medical record number, zip code, and type of patient

2. A health-care organization decides to buy a turnkey information system. The systems development life cycle phase that may be eliminated by doing this is the:
   A. Design phase
   B. Evaluation phase
   C. Implementation phase
   D. Research phase

3. Transcription services are provided by HIM department. An average of 30,000 lines of dictation are received each week. Minimum daily production for transcriptionists working 5 days per week is 1000 lines. Using the 15% adjustment factor to allow for vacation and sick days, the number of full-time employees needed to handle the transcription function is:
   A. 6.15
   B. 6.75
   C. 6.90
   D. 7.15

4. As part of a systems analysis process to design a record tracking system, the manager gathers information on the total number of medical records in the file and the number of locations in the organization where medical records may be used. This is part of the:
   A. Definition phase
   B. Design phase
   C. Feasibility phase
   D. Research phase

5. A health-care facility has made the decision to install an optical disk-based image/data management system. The following data are collected:

Number of inpatient records	146,000
Number of outpatient visits	320,000
Average number of pages/inpatient	37 pages
Average number of pages/outpatient	6 pages
Number of pages platter will hold	150,000

Using this information, the number of platters needed for these records is:

A. 13
B. 36
C. 49
D. 85

6. The computer system in place uses traditional file organization. Thus, many departments maintain their own information that cannot be accessed by others. To solve this problem, database management system software is being considered. This will result in:

A. Better data security
B. Ease in creating a database
C. Less data redundancy
D. Slower access

7. Computer workstations for six coders each use 60 square feet. Modular furniture would require only 36 square feet for each coder. Conversion to modular furniture would reduce the space requirement by:

A. 30%
B. 40%
C. 50%
D. 60%

8. A record processing unit adds diagnostic and procedure codes to the patient's computer record using mainframe terminals. When a code is entered the narrative for the code is not displayed. This problem is associated with:

A. Input
B. Processing
C. Output
D. Storage

9. The tumor registry contains 4800 records, each requiring an average of 2 kilobytes (K) of computer memory. One K = 1024 bytes and 1 megabyte (MB) = 1 million bytes. Storage of these records will require disk space of at least:

A. 5 MB
B. 10 MB
C. 15 MB
D. 20 MB

10. One way to monitor confidentiality of computer data is to attempt to obtain information for which you do not have authorization. This would be a monitor of:
    A. Backup system procedures
    B. Data misuse procedures
    C. Maintenancy procedures
    D. Recovery procedures

11. Smithville Clinic has recently installed a computerized patient record system. Several bills have been returned from insurance companies because the date of service had been omitted. The company representative confirmed that the software is capable of making the date of service a required field and not allowing the data entry person to leave the record until the date has been inserted. Such a measure to eliminate an omission is an example of:
    A. Data error correction
    B. Data error detection
    C. Data loss control
    D. Data misuse control

12. A large number of discharges have not been billed because of incomplete records. A computerized system that would be most likely to reduce the number of incomplete records is:
    A. Correspondence control system
    B. Database management system
    C. Master patient index system
    D. Record completion system

13. An electronic spreadsheet can manipulate health-care data, performing repeated calculations such as average daily census and percent of occupancy. Use of such software will:
    A. Decrease accuracy of data
    B. Increase accuracy of data
    C. Increase time needed to make calculations
    D. Ensure better use of data

14. The best software for determining budget variance is:
    A. Case-mix management system
    B. Database management system
    C. Spreadsheet package
    D. Word processing package

Stop MRT

15. In developing a request for proposal (RFP), instantaneous access to data is an example of:
    A. Constraint
    B. Objective
    C. Requirement
    D. User specification

Use the following information to answer questions 16 and 17:

Software for a release of information system was installed in January 1995. As manager of this unit, you are evaluating the system compared to the former system. You have gathered the following information:

	1994	1995
Average requests/month	210	245
Software license	$ 0	$ 1,200
Labor costs	$24,000	$12,000
Average fees charged/month	$ 1,500	$ 1,700
Average collections/month	$ 500	$ 1,200

16. Total direct costs as shown in the data collected have decreased by:
    A. 50%
    B. 51%
    C. 54%
    D. 57%

17. Further analysis of the data shows that the average cost per request for 1995 is:
  A. $48.90
  B. $24.50
  C. $12.25
  D. $ 4.08

Stop MRA

Answers and Explanations for Health Information Systems

1. **C.** *Level:* Problem solving   *Competency:* 1.3.1
   Rationale: Because you are specifying certain zip codes, a particular time period, and outpatients only, values for these fields must be identified in order to run the report.

2. **A** *Level:* Application   *Competency:* 3.1.6
   Source: Huffman (1994), page 495.

3. **C** *Level:* Problem solving   *Competency:* 2.2.6/2.2.1
   Rationale: $30{,}000/(1000 \times 5) = 6 \times 1.15 = 6.9$
   Source: Huffman (1994), pages 541–545.

4. **A** *Level:* Application   *Competency:* 2.1.8/2.1.5
   Source: Huffman (1994), pages 488–495.

5. **C** *Level:* Problem solving   *Competency:* 2.2.7/2.2.2
   Rationale: $(146{,}000 \times 37) + (320{,}000 \times 6)/150{,}000$
   Source: Huffman (1994), page 513.

6. **C** *Level:* Application   *Competency:* 2.1.16/2.1.6
   Source: Huffman (1994), pages 510–511.

7. **B** *Level:* Problem solving   *Competency:* 2.2.8/2.2.3
   Rationale: $60 - 36 = 24$ square feet saved $(24 \times 100)/60 = 40\%$
   Note: This is the same if calculated on one workstation or for all six workstations.

8. **C** *Level:* Application   *Competency:* 4.1.3/4.1.2
   Source: Huffman (1994), page 487.

9. **B** *Level:* Problem solving   *Competency:* 2.2.7/2.2.2
   Rationale: $4800 \times (2 \times 1024)/1{,}000{,}000 = 9.8$. Round up to 10.
   Source: Huffman (1994), page 502.

10. **B** *Level:* Application   *Competency:* 3.1.9
    Source: Huffman (1994), pages 562–563.

11. **B** *Level:* Application   *Competency:* 1.1.20/1.1.21
    Source: Huffman (1994), pages 558–562.

12. **D** *Level:* Application   *Competency:* 3.1.6
    Source: Huffman (1994), pages 533–539.

13. **B** *Level* Application   *Competency:* 1.2.5
    Rationale: By performing repeated calculations, mathematical errors will be reduced.
    Source: Huffman (1994), pages 537–539.

14. **B** *Level:* Application   *Competency:* 3.1.7
    Source: Huffman (1994), pages 537–539.

15. **C** *Level:* Application   *Competency:* 2.2.5
    Source: Huffman (1994), pages 492–493.

16. **B** *Level:* Problem Solving   *Competency:* 4.1.1
    Rationale: ($12,000 + $1,200) − $1,200/($24,000 − $500) = 51%

17. **D** *Level:* Problem solving   *Competency:* 4.1.1
    Rationale: ($12,000 + $1,200) − $1,200/(245 × 12) = $4.08

Health Information Systems References for Further Study

Ball, M. J., Douglas, J. V., O'Desky, R. I., & Albright, J. W. (Eds.). (1991). *Healthcare information management systems: A practical guide.* New York: Springer-Verlag.

Bourke, M. K. (1994). *The strategy and architecture of health care information systems.* New York: Springer-Verlag.

Drazen, E. L., Metzger, J. B., Ritter, J. L., & Schneider, M. K. (1995). *Patient care information systems: Successful design and implementation.* New York: Springer-Verlag.

FitzGerald, J., & FitzGerald, A. F. (1987). *Fundamentals of systems analysis: Using structured analysis and design techniques* (3rd ed.). New York: John Wiley & Sons.

Huffman, E. K. (1994). *Health information management* (10th ed.). Berwyn, IL: Physicians' Record Company.

Chapter 5

Health-Care Statistics

Overview

This chapter includes questions about descriptive statistics such as percentage of occupancy, average daily census, length of stay, and death and autopsy rates. Also included are questions about how to analyze and display health information in general.

The particular competencies that are tested in this chapter are listed below, both for MRAs and MRTs.

MRA Competencies

1.1.23 Abstract information from patient records (concurrently or retrospectively) for compilation of vital statistics.
1.2.1   Verify that data have been obtained from valid sources.
1.2.4   Check data for internal consistency.
1.3.1   Prepare data for analysis (i.e., compile data, develop graphs, tables, etc.).
1.3.8   Calculate institutional statistics (i.e., occupancy rates, census, length of stay).
1.3.9   Apply statistical techniques for analyzing departmental/institutional/patient-related data (i.e., mean, standard deviation, variance, etc.).

Chapter 5

MRT Competencies

1.1.24 Abstract information from patient records (concurrently or retrospectively) for compilation of vital statistics.
1.2.1 Verify that data have been obtained from valid sources.
1.2.4 Check data for internal consistency.
1.3.1 Prepare data for analysis (i.e., compile data, develop graphs, tables, etc.).
1.3.8 Calculate institutional statistics (i.e., occupancy rates, census, length of stay).
1.3.9 Apply statistical techniques for analyzing departmental/institutional/patient-related data (i.e., mean, standard deviation, variance, etc.).

Before you answer the questions, review your course material including all handouts, exercises, quizzes, and texts. Also review chapter 11 in *Health Information Management,* 10th edition (Huffman, 1994). Answering the questions in this chapter will help the reader review knowledge and skills about health-care statistics and analysis and display of data. Note: formulas are provided just before the test items. You may refer to these as you complete the questions in this chapter.

Use one of the answer sheets provided for Chapter 5 to record your answers. Choose the one best answer for each item. Mark either A, B, C, or D for each question number.

Again, be sure to show any problem solving you did, either beside the question in the review book or on a separate sheet of paper. This will help you retrace your steps and let you determine whether you made a careless error in math or reading. If you continue to make many of these kinds of errors, refer to Chapter 1 again, which reviews test-taking strategies. Also note if you had to guess at the answer by placing a question mark or other symbol beside the question. Guessing is an important clue that you may need more information about this topic.

After you answer the questions, check your choices against the answers and explanations provided. Use the number of questions that you answered correctly to calculate your score using the grid on the answer sheet. Again indicate those materials that you would like to review further before the national exam.

Place the score for this chapter on the separate grid that is provided. The grid will allow you to determine your overall score when you have completed all the tests. You will want to do further review in those areas where you record the lowest scores. References for study are provided at the end of the chapter.

Health-Care Formulas

Average Daily Census

$$\frac{\text{Total inpatient service days (exclude newborns) for a period}}{\text{Total number of days in the period}}$$

Average Length of Stay

$$\frac{\text{Total length of stay (discharge days) (include deaths; exclude newborns)}}{\text{Total discharges (include deaths; exclude newborns)}}$$

Percentage of Occupancy

$$\frac{\text{Daily inpatient census (inpatient service days, exclude newborns)} \times 100}{\text{Inpatient bed count} \times \text{days in the period}}$$

Hospital Death Rate

$$\frac{\text{Total inpatient deaths (include newborns)} \times 100}{\text{Total discharges (include deaths; include newborns)}}$$

Fetal Death Rate

$$\frac{\text{Total intermediate/late fetal deaths for a period} \times 100}{\text{Total live births + intermediate/late fetal deaths for the period}}$$

Gross Autospy Rate

$$\frac{\text{Total inpatient autopsies for a given period (include newborns)} \times 100}{\text{Total inpatient deaths for the period (include newborns)}}$$

Net Autopsy Rate

$$\frac{\text{Total inpatient autopsies for a given period (include newborns)} \times 100}{\text{Total inpatient deaths for the period (include newborns)} - \text{coroners' cases}}$$

Hospital Autopsy Rate (Adjusted)

$$\frac{\text{Total hospital autopsies for a given period} \times 100}{\text{Total deaths for the period whose bodies are available}}$$

Cesarean Section Rate

$$\frac{\text{Total number of c-sections performed in a period} \times 100}{\text{Total number of deliveries in the period (include c-sections)}}$$

Test Items

Health-Care Statistics Questions

Number of Items: 20
MRA Time Allowed: 18 minutes
MRT Time Allowed: 19 minutes

Start

1. The reliability of data refers to:
   A. Ability to measure what the data are intended to measure
   B. Repeatability of the data
   C. Representation of a normal distribution
   D. Source of the data

2. The percentage of occupancy for the newborn nursery for the year was 85.5%. There were 3121 patient days of care provided. The number of bassinets in this newborn nursery is:
   A. 8
   B. 10
   C. 15
   D. 20

3. In a 300-bed hospital, inpatient service days for April were 7392. The percentage of occupancy for April was:
   A. 70.2
   B. 73.9
   C. 82.1
   D. 84.6

4. A woman in the 27th week of pregnancy delivers a stillborn infant. This would be classified as:
   A. Infant death
   B. Early fetal death
   C. Intermediate fetal death
   D. Late fetal death

5. In August a hospital had 24 inpatient deaths with total discharges of 1291. The death rate for the month is:
   A. 0.02
   B. 0.19
   C. 1.86
   D. 2.19

6. A 200-bed facility had a 76.3% occupancy rate for 1994. The average daily census would be:
   A. 148
   B. 153
   C. 157
   D. 162

7. There were 121 inpatient deaths during 1994. Seven of these deaths were unautopsied medical examiner cases. Thirty-eight autopsies were performed by the hospital pathologists. The gross autopsy rate is:
   A. 25.6
   B. 27.2
   C. 31.4
   D. 33.3

8. A patient is admitted on July 28 and is discharged on August 15 of the same year. The length of stay for this patient is:
   A. 16 days
   B. 17 days
   C. 18 days
   D. 19 days

9. Data have been collected on patient satisfaction, grouped into categories of highly satisfied, satisfied, somewhat dissatisfied, and not satisfied at all. The most useful way to graphically display these data for analysis is a:
   A. Bar chart
   B. Flowchart
   C. Histogram
   D. Scattergram

10. A-175 bed hospital provided 3292 days of service to adults and children in September. The average daily census is:
   A. 88
   B. 101
   C. 110
   D. 119

11. During August, 823 patients were discharged and there were 5926 discharge days. The average length of stay for August is:
   A. 5.1 days
   B. 5.8 days
   C. 6.4 days
   D. 7.2 days

12. A table is needed to present demographic patient data to administration. The ages of patients range from less than 1 year to 92 years. The best way to group this datum is:
   A. 1–20
      21–40
      41–60
      61–80
   B. 0–14
      15–24
      25–34
      35–44
      45–54
      55–64
      65 & over
   C. 0–30
      31–60
      61–90
   D. 0–10
      10–20
      20–30
      30–40
      40–50
      50–60
      60 & over

44   Chapter 5

13. In 1994, a hospital had 125 deaths. There were 3 unautopsied medical examiner cases. Seventy-five inpatient autopies, as well as autopsies of 3 fetal deaths, were performed by the hospital pathology department. The net autopsy rate is:
    A. 60.6
    B. 61.5
    C. 62.4
    D. 63.9

14. You are reviewing the following table:

Patient Days by Age, First Quarter 1995, Hope Hospital

Age	Patients	Days	Percent
65 & over	75	1033	40.2
25–64	195	984	38.2
15–24	87	323	12.6
0–14	78	232	9.0

The age group with the least percent of patients is:
A. 65 & over
B. 25–64
C. 15–24
D. 0–14

15. During 1994, an average of 46 coronary artery bypass grafts (CABGs) were performed each month. Ten deaths occurred following this procedure in 1994. The death rate for CABGs is:
    A. 01.1%
    B. 01.8%
    C. 02.2%
    D. 21.7%

16. A medical staff committee has asked for all postoperative procedures grouped by procedure. A graph that is useful in presenting the proportion of deaths for a procedure in relation to all postoperative deaths is:

A. Bar chart
   B. Histogram
   C. Pie chart
   D. Scattergram

17. In 1994 there were 231 inpatient deaths. There were 120 autopsies performed on inpatients and 3 autopsies performed on former patients whose bodies were returned. There were 5 unautopsied medical examiner cases. The hospital autopsy rate (adjusted) is:
   A. 50.5%
   B. 51.9%
   C. 52.4%
   D. 53.7%

18. On June 1 the beginning census was 221. During the 24-hour census period there were 10 admissions and 12 discharges. Included in these admissions and discharges were 3 people who were both admitted and discharged. The census for June 2 is:
   A. 219
   B. 222
   C. 225
   D. 231

19. The length of stay for some patients is 3, 10, 1, 29, 4, 2, 6, 1, 4, and 5 days. The median stay for this group of patients is:
   A. 3.0 days
   B. 4.0 days
   C. 5.0 days
   D. 6.5 days

20. Length of stay data are being prepared for analysis. The best measure of the spread of these types of data is:
   A. Percentiles
   B. Range
   C. Standard deviation
   D. Variance

Stop

Answers and Explanations for Health-Care Statistics

1. **B** *Level:* Knowledge *Competency:* 1.2.1
   Source: Huffman (1994), page 449.

2. **B** *Level:* Problem solving *Competency:* 1.2.4
   Rationale: (3121/.855)/365 = 10 bassinets.
   This is a basic math procedure and allows you to check data for internal consistency.

3. **C** *Level:* Problem solving *Competency:* 1.3.8
   Rationale: $7392 \times 100 / 300 \times 30 = 82.1\%$
   Source: Hanken & Water (1994), pages 102–103.

4. **C** *Level:* Application *Competency:* 1.1.23/1.1.24
   Source: Hanken & Water (1994), pages 57–59.

5. **C** *Level:* Problem solving *Competency:* 1.3.8
   Rationale: $24 \times 100 / 1291 = 1.86$
   Source: Hanken & Water (1994), pages 105–106.

6. **B** *Level:* Problem solving *Competency:* 1.2.4
   Rationale: $200 \times .763 = 152.6$. Round to 153. You can multiply the percentage of occupancy times the bed capacity to compare to the average daily census and validate the internal consistency of the data.

7. **C** *Level:* Problem solving *Competency:* 1.3.8
   Rationale: $38 \times 100 / 121 = 31.4$
   Source: Hanken & Water (1994), pages 106–110.

8. **C** *Level:* Problem solving *Competency:* 1.3.8
   Rationale: $31 - 28 = 3$. $3 + 15 = 18$.
   Source: Hanken & Water (1994), pages 98–99.

9. **A** *Level:* Application *Competency:* 1.3.1
   Rationale: The bar chart works well with grouped data when the groups are characterized by nonnumerical attributes or categories.
   Source: Rosner (1990), page 28.

10. **C** *Level:* Problem solving *Competency:* 1.3.8
    Rationale: 3292/30 = 109.7. Round to 110.
    Source: Hanken & Water (1994), page 98.

11. **D** *Level:* Problem solving *Competency:* 1.3.8
    Rationale: 5926/823 = 7.2
    Source: Hanken & Water (1994), pages 99–101.

12. **B** *Level:* Application *Competency:* 1.3.1
    Rationale: Choice A does not cover all ages. Choice C has too few categories. Choice D categories are not mutually exclusive, i.e., you would not know where to place a person who is age 10.
    Source: Huffman (1994), pages 435–436.

13. **B** *Level:* Problem solving *Competency:* 1.3.8
    Rationale: $75 \times 100/(125 - 3) = 61.5\%$. Autopsies of fetal deaths are not included in reporting overall autopsy rates.
    Source: Hanken & Water (1994), pages 108–110.

14. **A** *Level:* Application *Competency:* 1.3.1
    Rationale: This group only had 75 of the 435 patients, or 17% (75/435). The question does not ask which group had the least percent of days.

15. **B** *Level:* Problem solving *Competency:* 1.3.8
    Rationale: $(10 \times 100)/(46 \times 12) = 1.8$
    Source: Hanken & Water (1994), pages 105–106.

16. **C** *Level:* Application *Competency:* 1.3.1
    Source: Huffman (1994), pages 436–440.

17. **D** *Level:* Problem solving *Competency:* 1.3.8
    Rationale: $(120 + 3) \times 100 (231 - 5) + 3 = 53.7$
    Source: Hanken & Water (1994), pages 108–110.

18. **A** *Level:* Problem solving *Competency:* 1.3.8
Rationale: 221 + 10 − 12 = 219
Source: Hanken & Water (1994), pages 96–98.

19. **B** *Level:* Problem solving *Competency:* 1.3.9
Rationale: When the data are arrayed in numerical order (1, 1, 2, 3, 4, 4, 5, 6, 10, 29) the center is between the two fours in this even number of cases. Therefore, (4 + 4)/2 = 4.
Source: Hanken & Water (1994), pages 90–93.

20. **C** *Level:* Application *Competency:* 1.3.9
Rationale: This measure tells us, on average, how much individual values differ from the mean. Because it relates so directly to the mean, it is the most widely used measure of variation in data.
Source: Norman & Streiner (1986), pages 23–24.

Health-Care Statistics References for Further Study

Duncan, R. C. (1983). *Introductory biostatistics for the health sciences* (2nd ed.). Albany, NY: Delmar Publishers, Inc.

Hanken, M., & Water, K. (1994). *Glossary of healthcare terms*. Chicago, IL: American Health Information Management Association.

Huffman, E. K. (1994). *Health information management* (10th ed.). Berwyn, IL: Physicians' Record Company.

Norman, G., & Streiner, D. (1986). *PDQ statistics*. Philiadelphia: B. C. Decker, Inc.

Pierce, P. (1987). *Commonly computed rates and percentages for hospital inpatients*. Chicago: American Health Information Management Association.

Rosner, B. (1990). *Fundamentals of biostatistics*. Boston: PWS-Kent Publishing Company.

Chapter 6

Quality of Health Care

Overview

This chapter covers utilization management, quality improvement, and risk management. Appropriate and efficient use of an organization's resources are the goals of utilization management. This function has been referred to as utilization review in the past and was begun in an effort to reduce the costs of health care. Quality improvement uses indicators to monitor the quality of care in a continuous and systematic way. There are many tools used in this process and an important focus is the trending of data. Risk management seeks to protect an organization from financial loss. Adverse events that create risk for the facility are important. Because these three functions are so closely related, it is useful to integrate the three processes.

The particular competencies that are tested in this chapter are listed below, both for MRAs and MRTs.

MRA Competencies

1.1.1 Conduct surveys of patients, users of data, health-care providers, administrators, and researchers.
1.1.2 Conduct interviews with users of data, health-care providers, administrators, researchers, and others.
1.1.4 Monitor changes in federal, state, and local laws, regulations, or Joint Commission standards.

1.1.10   Tabulate data on the appropriateness and quality of patient care as documented in the medical record (i.e., quality assurance, utilization review activities).
1.1.18   Design forms for collection of patient-related or other data (i.e., medical record forms, quality assurance, utilization review forms, etc.).
1.1.27   Participate in departmental or institutional committees.
1.3.5   Analyze employee performance data in relation to departmental/institutional performance standards.
1.3.6   Analyze physician performance data/profiles in relation to medical staff, institutional, or regulatory or accreditation standards.
1.3.7   Analyze clinical or institutional data in relation to previous or current internal and external patterns to identify trends and patterns.
2.1.1   Develop departmental plans, goals, and objectives for areas under your span of control.
2.1.20   Develop in-service education programs for departmental or nondepartmental staff.
3.1.5   Monitor adherence to system specification.
3.1.15   Conduct educational programs for departmental or nondepartmental staff.
4.1.3   Recommend changes or improvement(s) in systems.

MRT Competencies

1.1.1   Conduct surveys of patients, users of data, health-care providers, administrators, and researchers.
1.1.2   Conduct interviews with users of data, health-care providers, administrators, researchers, and others.
1.1.4   Monitor changes in federal, state, and local laws, regulations, or Joint Commission standards.
1.1.10   Tabulate data on the appropriateness and quality of patient care as documented in the medical record (i.e., quality assurance, utilization review activities).
1.1.19   Design forms for collection of patient-related or other data (i.e., medical record forms, quality assurance, utilization review forms, etc.).
1.1.29   Participate in departmental or institutional committees.

1.3.4   Analyze employee performance data in relation to departmental/institutional performance standards.
2.1.1   Develop departmental plans, goals, and objectives for areas under your span of control.
2.1.20   Develop in-service education programs for departmental or nondepartmental staff.
3.1.5   Monitor adherence to system specification.
3.1.15   Conduct educational programs for departmental or nondepartmental staff.
4.1.2   Recommend changes or improvement(s) in systems.

Before you answer the questions, review your course material including all handouts, exercises, quizzes, and texts. Also review chapter 16 in *Health Information Management,* 10th edition (Huffman 1994). Answering the questions in this chapter will help the reader review knowledge and skills used in the assessment of quality in health.

Use one of the answer sheets provided for Chapter 6 to record your answers. Choose the one best answer for each item. Mark either A, B, C, or D for each question number.

Again, be sure to show any problem solving you did, either beside the question in the review book or on a separate sheet of paper. This will help you retrace your steps and let you determine whether you made a careless error in math or reading. If you continue to make many of these kinds of errors, refer to Chapter 1 again, which reviews test-taking strategies. Also note if you had to guess at the answer by placing a question mark or other symbol beside the question. Guessing is an important clue that you may need more information about this topic.

After you answer the questions, check your choices against the answers and explanations provided. Use the number of questions that you answered correctly to calculate your score using the grid on the answer sheet. Again indicate those materials that you would like to review further before the national exam.

Place the score for this chapter on the separate grid that is provided. The grid will allow you to determine your overall score when you have completed all the tests. You will want to do further review in those areas where you record the lowest scores. References for study are provided at the end of the chapter.

Chapter 6

Test Items

Quality of Health-Care Questions

Number of Items: 20 MRA/19 MRT (Omit last question)
MRA Time Allowed: 18 minutes
MRT Time Allowed: 18 minutes

Start

1. A department quality inspection team has identified the likely cause of a problem and has decided on a course of action to correct this problem. The team decides at this point to use a quality improvement tool that focuses on one problem and then tests a solution. The team will use:
   A. Cause and effect diagram
   B. Pareto chart
   C. PDCA method
   D. Satisfaction survey

2. You are assisting the Department of Internal Medicine as it develops its quality improvement plan. Critical indicators are being developed for the department. A CPK above normal range and associated with an abnormal ECG is an indicator example of:
   A. Appropriateness
   B. Intensity of service
   C. Severity of illness
   D. Volume

3. JCAHO, in its 10-step procedure, requires that a hospital's quality program concentrate on:
   A. Collecting and organizing data
   B. Creating a QI committee
   C. Creating a list of problems
   D. Studying specific diseases

4. The contract between Health Care Financing Administration (HCFA) and the Professional Review Organizations (PROs) is called the:
   A. HCFA contract
   B. Medicare Conditions of Participation
   C. Memorandum of Understanding
   D. PRO Scope of Work

5. A department manager forms a QI team to work on the problem of diagnostic reports that have not been filed in patient records. First, the group decides to look for possible causes for this problem. An appropriate tool for this group to use would be:
   A. Cause and effect diagram
   B. Flowchart
   C. Pareto chart
   D. Scatter diagram

6. A mail survey of the customers of the health information management functions is being planned. When designing the questionnaire that will be used it is important to:
   A. Include as many questions as possible
   B. Only send the form to those who are happy with the services provided
   C. Use open-ended questions
   D. Use a cordial, helpful, and polite tone

Use the following information to answer questions 7 through 10:

Coding Errors Related to Principal Diagnosis by Coder, First Quarter, 1995

	Coders						
	LB	AD	JE	SJ	DS	RW	Total
Wrong Code Sequence OK	0	2	3	4	4	12	25
Sequence Wrong Code OK	17	3	4	0	0	0	24
Principal Dx Missing	5	0	0	0	3	4	12
Sequence and Code Wrong	1	0	0	0	0	0	1
Total	23	5	7	4	7	16	62

7. In analyzing the information collected in a department's QI program you find two types of problems result in the majority of errors for the coding function. These errors as shown in the table are:
    A. Wrong code but sequence correct/Correct code but sequence wrong
    B. Wrong code but sequence correct/Principal diagnosis missing
    C. Correct code but sequence wrong/Sequence and code wrong
    D. Correct code but sequence wrong/Principal diagnosis missing

8. Two coders are responsible for a majority of the principal diagnosis coding errors. These coders are:
    A. LB and AD
    B. JE and RW
    C. SJ and LB
    D. RW and LB

9. The most economical course of action to quickly reduce the most errors is:
    A. Hire a coding consultant
    B. Provide basic coding training for all coders
    C. Provide training on sequencing to LB
    D. Send all coders to an advanced coding workshop

10. One of the best tools for analyzing the data shown in the table is a:
    A. Check sheet
    B. Flowchart
    C. Pareto chart
    D. Run chart

11. A hospital committee wants a form designed for use in gathering data from patients about their level of satisfaction with the organization. The data elements have been determined and, as director of HIM (Health Information Management), you have been asked to produce a master form for the committee to review in 2 weeks. The fastest and most economical way to produce a well designed form is to:
    A. Use desktop publishing software
    B. Consult a forms design company
    C. Use a spreadsheet
    D. Consult a typesetting company

12. The manager of a quality improvement department determines that information to improve patient care is needed more quickly. After reviewing the process, the manager decides that data should be collected during patient hospitalization. This is:

A. Admission review
B. Concurrent review
C. Preadmission review
D. Retrospective review

13. A hospital interviews patients about their satisfaction with its services. This information is communicated to the risk manager. Use of these data would be part of the component of risk management called:
    A. Risk assessment
    B. Risk control
    C. Risk financing
    D. Risk identification

14. A physician advisor has decided that a certain Medicare patient is not eligible for further care. The attending physician agrees with this decision. The next step is to:
    A. Discharge the patient immediately
    B. Notify the patient, the business office, the attending physician, and the PRO
    C. Have the UR committee meet
    D. Have the UR coordinator visit and notify the patient

Use the following information to answer questions 15 and 16:

As manager of the Utilization Management Section, you have compiled the following report of admission denials by the Professional Review Organization (PRO) for the past 2 years.

Hope Hospital Admission Denials by PRO

Reason for Review	1994 Denials Number (%)	1995 Denials Number (%)
3% Random Sample	34 (1.9%)	29 (1.5%)
Transfers	10 (1.0%)	10 (0.9%)
Readmissions (31 Days)	45 (1.3%)	75 (2.1%)
Beneficiary Complaints	5 (5.5%)	4 (4.8%)
Focused DRGs	18 (0.24%)	13 (0.19%)

15. Review of the information shows that the area that needs further study is:
    A. Beneficiary complaints
    B. Focused DRGs
    C. Readmissions
    D. Transfers

16. As manager of the utilization management function you serve on the Utilization Management Committee of the medical staff. You decide that the best course of action would be to:
    A. Consult with the chairperson of the UM Committee
    B. Do nothing because this is a medical staff issue
    C. Present the report at the next UM Committee meeting
    D. Refer the matter to administration without involving the UM Committee

17. As director of HIM Services you are developing an in-service program on quality improvement for the department employees. The first step you should take in preparing for the in-service is to:
    A. Create slides or overheads for the presentation
    B. Decide on a date and time for the session
    C. Develop objectives for the presentation
    D. Schedule use of the conference room for the session

18. The Quality Management Committee has historically excluded the HIM department manager. The HIM manager asks for an appointment to this committee. She points out her training would be an asset in all the following activities except:
    A. Data gathering
    B. Developing criteria or indicators
    C. Displaying data
    D. Providing resources for criteria development

19. Data collection is an important part of assessing quality, risk, and utilization of an organization. One of the best ways to improve the quality of data and to minimize employee time is to
    A. Integrate the data collection processes
    B. Use only RNs to collect data
    C. Use only RRAs or ARTs to collect data
    D. Use both RNs and RRAs/ARTs to collect data

Stop MRT

20. Dr. Brown applies for appointment to the medical staff. After review of his license, education, postgraduate training, experience, and disciplinary actions, the medical staff recommends his appointment to the governing board. This process is:
    A. Credentialing
    B. Profiling
    C. Risk management
    D. Utilization review

Stop MRA

Answers and Explanations for Quality of Health Care

1. **C** *Level:* Application *Competency:* 4.1.3/4.1.2
   Source: Cofer & Greeley (1992), pages 79–84.

2. **C** *Level:* Application *Competency:* 1.1.10
   Source: Huffman (1994), pages 628–631.

3. **A** *Level:* Application *Competency:* 1.1.4
   Source: Huffman (1994), page 610.

4. **D** *Level:* Application *Competency:* 1.1.4
   Source: Huffman (1994), page 623.

5. **A** *Level:* Application *Competency:* 2.1.1
   Source: Cofer & Greeley (1992), pages 50–52.

6. **D** *Level:* Application *Competency:* 1.1.1
   Source: Cofer & Greeley (1992), pages 39–44.

7. **A** *Level:* Application *Competency:* 1.3.5/1.3.4
   Rationale: Wrong code but sequence correct accounts for 40.3% of the errors. Correct code but sequence wrong comprises 38.7% of the errors. 40.3 + 38.7 = 79%.

8. **D** *Level:* Application *Competency:* 1.3.5/1.3.4
   Rationale: RW is responsible for 25.3% of the errors, LB for 37.1%. 25.3 + 37.1 = 62.4%.

9. **C** *Level:* Problem solving *Competency:* 2.1.20/2.1.7
   Rationale: Providing training for the one coder who is responsible for 37% of the errors has the potential of reducing errors by over one-third. Obviously LB is a good coder and primarily has a problem with determining the principal diagnosis.

10. **C** *Level:* Application *Competency:* 1.3.5/1.3.4
    Source: Cofer & Greeley (1992), pages 60–63.

Quality of Health Care 59

11. **A** *Level:* Problem solving   *Competency:* 1.1.18/1.1.19

    Rationale: Consulting a forms design company or a typesetting company is neither cheap nor fast when developing forms. Spreadsheet software is not suitable for developing forms; however, desktop publishing software would allow for this task to be done quite well.

    Source: Huffman (1994), pages 537–539.

12. **B** *Level:* Application   *Competency:* 4.1.3/4.1.2

    Source: Huffman (1994), pages 405, 628.

13. **D** *Level:* Application   *Competency:* 1.1.2

    Source: Huffman (1994), pages 637–639.

14. **B** *Level:* Application   *Competency:* 3.1.5

    Source: Huffman (1994), pages 627–628.

15. **C** *Level:* Problem solving   *Competency:* 1.3.7/1.1.10

    Rationale: The only type of review that has resulted in an increase in percentage of denials is readmission within 31 days. This is a finding that would warrant further study to determine causes and identify potential problems. Although there was an increase in the number of denials in the 3% random sample, the percentage actually dropped.

16. **A** *Level:* Problem solving   *Competency:* 1.1.27/1.1.29

    Rationale: The best choice is to consult with the chair of the Utilization Management Committee and allow that person to decide the best method for dealing with this potential problem. It is not appropriate to refer the matter to administration without involving the chair of the Utilization Management Committee who has been given responsibility for ensuring that the utilization of the facility's resources by the medical staff is appropriate. To do nothing is not in the organization's best interests. Presenting the report at the next UM Committee meeting will result in further delays in dealing with this problem.

17. **C** *Level:* Application   *Competency:* 3.1.15

    Source: Cofer & Greeley (1992), pages 169–172.

18. **B** *Level:* Application   *Competency:* 4.1.3/4.1.2

    Rationale: Only the individuals providing the clinical services (e.g., physicians, nurses, physical therapists, etc.) can develop indicators or criteria on which to evaluate those services received by a patient. Professionals trained in health information do have the skills to provide all the other services to these groups.

19. **A** *Level:* Application   *Competency:* 4.1.3/4.1.2

    Source: Mangano (1993), pages 154–156.
    Huffman (19940, pages 609, 627.

20. **A** *Level:* Application   *Competency:* 1.3.6

    Source: Huffman (1994), pages 631–635.

Quality of Health-Care References for Further Study

Ciccone, K., & Lord, J. (1992). *IQA-2: Continuous performance improvement through integrated quality assessment.* Chicago, IL: American Hospital Association.

Cofer, J., & Greeley, H. (1992). *Quality improvement techniques for medical records: A handbook.* Marblehead, MA: Opus Communications.

Huffman, E. K. (1994). *Health information management* (10th edition). Berwyn, IL: Physicians' Record Company.

Joint Commission on Accreditation of Healthcare Organizations. (1991). *Using quality improvement tools in a health care setting.* Chicago, IL: Joint Commission on Accreditation of Healthcare Organizations.

Joint Commission on Accreditation of Healthcare Organizations (1993). *The measurement mandate.* Chicago, IL: Joint Commission on Accreditation of Healthcare Organizations.

Joint Commission on Accreditation of Healthcare Organizations (1994). *1995 Accreditation manual for hospitals. Volume I: Standards.* Chicago, IL: Joint Commission on Accreditation of Healthcare Organizations.

Spath, P. (1991). *Health care quality: A practical guide to continuous improvement.* Forest Grove, OR: Brown-Spath & Associates.

Chapter **7**

Classification Systems

Overview

This chapter deals with the systems for classifying and recording disease information. In order to identify and classify disease processes, a standardized system must be used. There are many nomenclatures and classification systems. This chapter is primarily concerned with CPT-4, DSM-IV, and ICD-9-CM. Some common reimbursement issues are also included in this chapter.

The particular competencies that are tested in this chapter are listed below, both for MRAs and MRTs.

MRA Competencies

- 1.1.7 Compare claims submitted to third-party payers with reimbursement received.
- 1.1.29 Assign diagnostic/procedure codes using ICD-9-CM, CPT, HCPCS, DSM, or other coding systems.
- 1.2.7 Validate diagnostic and procedure coding (i.e., ICD-9-CM, CPT, HCPCS, or other coding systems).
- 1.3.2 Perform departmental/institutional case-mix analysis.
- 1.3.11 Analyze case-mix payment rates (i.e, DRG and others) to determine reimbursement optimization.

62 *Chapter 7*

MRT Competencies

1.1.7 Compare claims submitted to third-party payers with reimbursement received.
1.1.31 Assign diagnostic/procedure codes using ICD-9-CM, CPT, HCPCS, DSM, or other coding systems.
1.2.7 Validate diagnostic and procedure coding (i.e., ICD-9-CM, CPT, HCPCS, or other coding systems).
1.3.2 Perform departmental/institutional case-mix analysis.
1.3.6 Analyze case-mix payment rates (i.e, DRG and others) to determine reimbursement optimization.

Before you answer the questions, review your course material including all handouts, exercises, quizzes, and texts. Also review chapters 9 and 12 in *Health Information Management,* 10th edition(Huffman 1994). Answering the questions in this chapter will help the reader review knowledge and skills needed to properly use health-care classification systems.

Use one of the answer sheets provided for Chapter 7 to record your answers. Choose the one best answer for each item. Mark either A, B, C, or D for each question number.

Again, be sure to show any problem solving you did, either beside the question in the review book or on a separate sheet of paper. This will help you retrace your steps and let you determine whether you made a careless error in math or reading. If you continue to make many of these kinds of errors, refer to Chapter 1 again, which reviews test-taking strategies. Also note if you had to guess at the answer by placing a question mark or other symbol beside the question. Guessing is an important clue that you may need more information about this topic.

After you answer the questions, check your choices against the answers and explanations provided. Use the number of questions that you answered correctly to calculate your score using the grid on the answer sheet. Again indicate those materials that you would like to review further before the national exam.

Place the score for this chapter on the separate grid that is provided. The grid will allow you to determine your overall score when you have completed all the tests. You will want to do further review in those areas where you record the lowest scores. References for study are provided at the end of the chapter.

Test Items

Classification Systems Questions

Number of Items: 20
MRA Time Allowed: 18 minutes
MRT Time Allowed: 19 minutes

Start

1. The multiaxial system, DSM-IV, is used in facilities that provide specialized services for:
   A. Ambulatory patients
   B. OB-gynecological patients
   C. Pediatric patients
   D. Psychiatric patients

2. Which of the following is an acceptable eponym for coding a diagnosis:
   A. Arthrotomy of knee joint
   B. Plastic operation of arm with full-thickness skin graft
   C. Laennec's cirrhosis
   D. Urticaria/hives

3. HCFA's Common Procedure Coding System (HCPCS) is used to obtain reimbursement for:
   A. All care to Medicaid patients
   B. Hospital laboratory and pathology services
   C. Primary-care encounters and visits
   D. Part B (physician services) of Medicare

4. *Current Procedural Terminology*, 4th edition (CPT-4), is published and updated by:
   A. American Medical Association
   B. American Health Information Management Association
   C. Joint Commission on Accreditation of Healthcare Organizations
   D. American Hospital Association

5. Of the following ICD-9-CM codes, the one that can be used as principal diagnosis is:
   A. V27.0 Outcome of delivery, single liveborn
   B. E966 Assault by cutting and piercing instrument
   C. V30.00 Single liveborn, born in hospital
   D. M9010/0 Fibroadenoma, NOS

6. The effects a person experiences when there is an interaction between two or more prescribed drugs, taken as directed, may be classified in ICD-9-CM as a/an:
   A. Accidental poisoning
   B. Adverse effect
   C. Homicide attempt
   D. Late effect

7. In the diagnostic statement "acute and chronic bronchitis," the terms coded are:
   A. "Acute" only
   B. "Chronic" only
   C. Whichever occurred first
   D. Both "acute" and "chronic"

Use the following information to answer questions 8 and 9:

A 72-year-old patient was admitted to the hospital with chest pains. Tests indicated the presence of an acute inferior wall myocardial infarction. Five days after the admission the patient was found to have a lesion on the lung suspicious of carcinoma. The patient underwent a needle biopsy of the lesion and was discharged home 3 days later.

8. The patient's principal diagnosis is:
   A. Chest pain
   B. Carcinoma of lung
   C. Acute inferior wall myocardial infarction
   D. Lesion of lung

9. A comorbid condition present on this admission was:
   A. Chest pains
   B. Myocardial infarction
   C. Lesion of lung
   D. Senile dementia

10. A coding supervisor is reviewing records for correct DRG assignment based on complete coding of the clinical information. She is particularly interested in knowing if comorbid conditions or complications are being omitted in the coding process. The table below shows the findings of this review.

DRG 80: Respiratory Infect, Age >17, W/O CC

Coder#	Records Coded#	With CC Present
Baker	59	5
Davis	82	6
Johnson	25	3
White	48	4

The employee having the highest percent of incorrectly coded records resulting in the wrong DRG assignment is:

A. Baker
B. Davis
C. Johnson
D. White

11. A condition that arises during the hospital stay that prolongs the patient's length of stay by at least 1 day in 75% of the cases is the:

A. Principal diagnosis
B. Admitting diagnosis
C. Comorbidity
D. Complication

12. In referring to topography, one is referring to:

A. Cause of disease
B. Anatomical site
C. Pyramid placement
D. Histology

13. The condition established, after study, to be chiefly responsible for occasioning the admission of the patient to the hospital for care is the:

A. Primary diagnosis
B. Provisional diagnosis
C. Principal diagnosis
D. Major diagnosis

14. When given a differential diagnosis (e.g., acute pancreatitis vs. acute cholecystitis) the coder should code:
    A. Both diagnoses
    B. Neither diagnosis
    C. Only the diagnosis that is clearly documented
    D. Only the diagnosis that uses the most resources

15. Ms. Jones is seen in the hospital ambulatory surgery unit. She has been diagnosed with colonic polyps and undergoes a colonoscopy with biopsy. In your position as medical records coder for the hospital you would use the following codes:
    A. ICD-9-CM codes only
    B. ICD-9-CM codes and CPT codes
    C. CPT codes only
    D. ICD-9-CM and HCPCS codes

16. The chief financial officer of your facility has asked you to change code numbers to increase reimbursement for a patient. You review the record and determine that the documentation does not support the change of codes. Your best course of action is to:
    A. Do what he tells you to do
    B. Discuss the issue with the attending physician
    C. Tactfully inform him of your ethical and professional responsibilities
    D. Listen to him but do what you feel is the right thing to do

17. As supervisor of the coding section you have been requested to update and revise the hospital's coding guidelines. You include that for reporting to third-party payers, the sequence of codes should be according to definitions in the
    A. AHA Coding Clinics
    B. ICD-9-CMP
    C. UB-92
    D. UHDDS

18. Your facility's dollar rate is $3500. If a patient at your facility is assigned to a DRG with a case weight of .5010, the DRG payment would be:
    A. $ 508.00
    B. $1753.50
    C. $3500.00
    D. $6986.00

Use the information in the following table to answer questions 19 and 20:

XYZ Hospital
Descriptive Case Mix Report
Summary of Length of Stay by DRG

MDC 1: Diseases and Disorders of the Nervous System

DRG #	Cases	Mean	Total Days	Low	High
4	3	11.7	35	5	41
6	80	2.5	199	1	5
7	8	22.5	178	1	41
8	29	2.4	70	1	8
9	6	14.2	85	2	44
10	7	27.3	191	2	46
11	5	17.0	85	2	24
12	45	35.4	1591	2	48
13	7	15.4	108	2	30
14	223	31.2	6968	2	41
	413	23.0	9510		

19. Which DRG represents the highest average length of stay?
    A. 12
    B. 10
    C. 8
    D. 14

20. Which DRG represents one-fifth of the total cases for MDC 1?
    A. 6
    B. 8
    C. 12
    D. 14

Stop

Answers and Explanations for Classification Systems

1. **D** *Level:* Knowledge *Competency:* 1.1.29/1.1.31
   Source: Huffman (1994), pages 342–344

2. **C** *Level:* Application *Competency:* 1.2.7
   Source: Basic ICD-9-CM Coding Rules.

3. **D** *Level:* Knowledge *Competency:* 1.1.29/1.1.31
   Source: Huffman (1994), page 361.

4. **A** *Level:* Knowledge *Competency:* 1.1.29/1.1.31
   Source: Huffman (1994), pages 329–331.

5. **C** *Level:* Application *Competency:* 1.2.7
   Source: Basic ICD-9-CM Coding Rules.

6. **B** *Level:* Knowledge *Competency:* 1.1.29/1.1.31
   Source: Basic ICD-9-CM Coding Rules.

7. **D** *Level:* Application *Competency:* 1.1.29/1.1.31
   Source: AHA Official Guideline 1.4.

8. **C** *Level:* Application *Competency:* 1.1.29/1.1.31
   Source: AHA Official Guideline 2.

9. **C** *Level:* Application *Competency:* 1.1.29/1.1.31
   Source: AHA Official Guideline 3.

10. **C** *Level:* Application *Competency:* 1.3.11/1.3.6
    Rationale: The employee who has the highest percentage of records that had a complication or comorbid condition present and did not code this condition is Johnson. $3 \times 100 / 25 = 12\%$.

11. **D** *Level:* Knowledge *Competency:* 1.1.29/1.1.31
    Source: Uniform Hospital Discharge Data Set.
    Huffman (1994), pages 398–400.

12. **B** *Level:* Knowledge *Competency:* 1.1.29/1.1.31
    Source: Huffman (1994), page 325.

13. **C** *Level:* Knowledge *Competency:* 1.1.29/1.1.31
    Source: Huffman (1994), pages 378–400.

14. **A** *Level:* Application *Competency:* 1.2.7
    Source: AHA Official Guidelines 2.6.

15. **B** *Level:* Application *Competency:* 1.2.7
    Source: Guidelines for reporting of Ambulatory Services.

16. **C** *Level:* Application *Competency:* 1.2.7
    Source: Huffman (1994), pages 470–475.

17. **D** *Level:* Application *Competency:* 1.2.7
    Source: Huffman (1994), page 339.

18. **B** *Level:* Application *Competency:* 1.3.11
    Rationale: $3500 \times .5010 = $1753.50

19. **A** *Level:* Application *Competency:* 1.3.2
    Rationale: The highest average length of stay is represented by DRG 12 with an ALOS of 35.4.

20. **A** *Level:* Application *Competency:* 1.3.2
    Rationale: DRG 6, with 80 cases, represents approximately one-fifth of the total 413 cases for MDC 1.

Classification Systems References for Further Study

American Hospital Association. *Official ICD-9-CM coding guidelines for coding and reporting.* Chicago: American Hospital Association.

Brown, F. (1994). *ICD-9-CM coding handbook* (1994 revised ed.). American Hospital Association Publishing.

Huffman, E. K. (1994). *Health information management* (10th ed.). Berwyn, IL: Physicians' Record Company.

Nicholas, Toula (1995). *Basic ICD-9-CM coding handbook.* Chicago: American Health Information Management Association.

Nicholas, Toula (1995). *CPT/HCPCS basic coding handbook.* Chicago: American Health Information Management Association.

Chapter 8

Coding

Overview

This chapter deals with ICD-9-CM and CPT-4 coding problems. Ideally, when assigning codes you would use the entire record to help you make the best choice. For this review, as for AHIMA's national certifying examinations, you will use the information provided in each question.

There are only two competencies that are tested in this chapter. These competencies, for both MRAs and MRTs, are listed below.

MRA Competencies

1.1.29 Assign diagnostic/procedure codes using ICD-9-CM, CPT, HCPCS, DSM, or other coding systems.
1.2.7 Validate diagnostic and procedure coding (i.e., ICD-9-CM, CPT, HCPCS, or other coding systems).

MRT Competencies

1.1.31 Assign diagnostic/procedure codes using ICD-9-CM, CPT, HCPCS, DSM, or other coding systems.
1.2.7 Validate diagnostic and procedure coding (i.e., ICD-9-CM, CPT, HCPCS, or other coding systems).

Before you answer the questions, review your course material including all handouts, exercises, quizzes, and texts or workbooks that you used in your coding classes. Make sure your review includes the basic ICD-9-CM coding rules and the AHA Official Coding Guidelines. Answering the questions in this chapter will help the reader review knowledge and skills used for correctly coding patient records using ICD-9-CM and CPT-4.

Use one of the answer sheets provided for Chapter 8 to record your answers. Choose the one best answer for each item. Mark either A, B, C, or D for each question number.

Be sure to note if you had to guess at the answer by placing a question mark or other symbol beside the question. Guessing is an important clue that you may need more information about this area of coding.

After you answer the questions, check your choices against the answers and explanations provided. Use the number of questions that you answered correctly to calculate your score using the grid on the answer sheet. Note if you have problems with a particular coding rule or official guideline. Again indicate those materials that you would like to review further before the national exam.

Place the score for this chapter on the separate grid that is provided. The grid will allow you to determine your overall score when you have completed all the tests. You will want to do further review in those areas where you record the lowest scores. References for study are provided at the end of the chapter.

Note: you may use your ICD-9-CM and CPT-4 code books as you answer these questions.

Chapter 8

Test Items

Coding Questions

Number of Items: 30
MRA Time Allowed: 90 minutes
MRT Time Allowed: 90 minutes

Start

Use the following information to answer questions 1 through 10:

As part of the quality control for clinical information you have had the four clinical analysts assign ICD-9-CM codes for several patients.

1. Mrs. Phillips is a 65-year-old patient with severe diverticulitis of the transverse colon. She is admitted to the hospital and surgery is performed. The procedures listed on the face sheet of the record include creation of temporary ileostomy and resection of portion of transverse colon with end-to-end anastomosis. The following codes were assigned by the four coders. The appropriate codes for Mrs. Phillips are:

   A. 562.11, 45.74, 46.21
   B. 562.11, 45.74, 46.21, 45.94
   C. 751.5, 45.74, 46.21
   D. 562.11, 45.74, 45.94

2. Mr. Frank Jones was admitted with an acute myocardial infarction. The history and physical denotes the following additional diagnoses: status post cholecystectomy, status post aortocornary bypass, nevus on right arm, and blindness. The correct code(s) for Mr. Jones (is) are:

   A. 410.90
   B. 410.90, 216.9, 369.00
   C. 410.90, V45.81, 369.00
   D. 410.90, V45.89, 369.00

3. An 82-year-old female is admitted with a diagnosis of septicemia with shock. Blood cultures reveal staphylococcus. The correct codes would be:
   A. 038.9, 041.10, 785.59
   B. 041.10, 038.9
   C. 038.1, 785.59
   D. 038.0, 785.59

4. The clinical resume lists the final diagnosis for a 76-year-old male as congestive heart failure, acute pulmonary edema, hypertension, diabetes mellitus. The following codes were assigned by the four coders. The appropriate codes for this patient are:
   A. 428.0, 518.4, 401.9, 250.00
   B. 402.91, 518.4, 401.9, 250.00
   C. 428.0, 401.9, 250.00
   D. 402.91, 250.00

5. A 65-year-old male has carcinoma of the left lower lobe of the lung with metastasis to the bone. The patient is anemic and admitted for transfusions of 2 units of packed red blood cells. The diagnoses would be sequenced as:
   A. 162.5, 198.5, 285.9
   B. 285.9, 162.5, 198.5
   C. 198.5, 162.5, 285.9
   D. 285.9, 198.5, 162.5

6. A passenger on a motorcycle suffered compound fractures of right superior and inferior maxilla due to a collision with a car. Open reduction of mandible with internal fixation and open reduction of maxilla with alloplastic implant were performed. The following codes were assigned by the four coders. The appropriate codes for these injuries are:
   A. 802.4, E812.2, 76.74, 76.76
   B. 802.20, 802.4, E812.2, 76.74, 76.76
   C. 802.5, 802.30, E812.3, 76.76, 76.74, 76.92
   D. 802.28, 802.4, E812.3, 76.76, 76.74, 76.92

7. Pregnancy at term spontaneously delivered vaginally single liveborn. Midline episiotomy with repair. Patient has history of previous cesarean section. The appropriate codes for this patient are:
   A. 650, V27.0, 73.6
   B. 650, 73.6
   C. 654.23, V27.0, 73.6
   D. 654.21, V27.0, 76.3

8. A patient with brain damage, which is a late effect of cerebral anoxia due to barbiturate overdose. The patient made a suicide attempt 1 year ago. The appropriate codes for this patient are:
   A. 997.0, 909.0, 967.0
   B. 349.9, 995.2, 909.4, E950.1
   C. 348.1, 909.0, E959
   D. 997.0, 967.0, E950.1

9. Mr. Walter Anderson, who has carcinoma of the lung hilus, was admitted for infusion of chemotherapy. This record should be coded as:
   A. V58.1, 99.25
   B. 162.2, V58.1, 99.25
   C. V58.9, 262.2, 99.25
   D. V58.1, 162.2, 99.25

10. A 35-year-old patient was admitted to hospital with pneumonia due to *Pneumocystis carinii* and AIDS. The following codes were assigned by the four coders. The appropriate codes for this patient are:
    A. 136.3, 042
    B. 042, 482.9
    C. 482.9, 042
    D. 042, 136.3

11. Hemiplegia secondary to cerebral thrombosis (8 months ago) would be accurately coded as:
    A. 342.90, 436
    B. 434.0, 342.90
    C. 342.90, 438
    D. 433.9, 342.9

12. Mrs. Mattie Cohen, age 75, has been a diabetic for 20 years. For the past 5 years, the patient has been maintained on 50 units of NPH 100 insulin. Diagnosis: intercapillary glomerulosclerosis, peripheral angiopathy (diabetic), diabetes mellitus. The appropriate codes for this patient are:
    A. 250.81, 581.81, 443.81
    B. 250.40, 250.70, 581.81, 443.81
    C. 581.81, 443.81, 250.40, 250.70
    D. 250.41, 250.71, 581.81, 443.81

13. Rosie Gonzalez was admitted to the ambulatory surgery unit for a flexor tenotomy for three fingers of the left hand. The appropriate code(s) for this patient (is) are:
    A. 26450
    B. 26455, 26455, 26455
    C. 26460
    D. 26460, 26460, 26460

14. The clinical resume final diagnostic statement reads: "Acute upper respiratory infection, diabetes mellitus." The medication record includes Keflex, Beconase Spray, Diabinese, and Tolectin. The diagnosis that you would ask the physician to add to the physician statement is:
    A. Arthritis
    B. Headache
    C. Hypertension
    D. Phlebitis

15. Ms. Randolph was admitted to the hospital with coughing, SOB, and greenish purulent sputum. She also had 2+ pitting edema with a temperature of 102°F. Chest x-ray showed infiltrate in left lower lobe with some changes consistent with congestive heart failure. Sputum culture grew *Escherichia coli* sensitive to Rocephin. The patient was treated with Lasix and Rocephin. She has a history of hypertension and was continued on her hypertension medication during her stay. The appropriate sequence of diagnoses would be:
    A. 428.0, 482.82, 401.9
    B. 482.82, 428.0, 401.9
    C. 401.9, 482.82, 428.0
    D. 428.0, 486, 041.4

16. Betty Brown admitted with third-degree burns on the left arm and chest, second- and third-degree burns on the abdomen and left leg due to a house fire. Fifty percent of the body surface is burned, 20% at third degree. The appropriate codes are:
    A. 943.30, 942.32, 942.33, 945.30, 948.52, E890.3
    B. 942.39, 943.30, 945.30, 948.52, E890.3
    C. 942.30, 943.30, 945.30, 948.25, E890.9
    D. 942.32, 942.33, 943.30, 945.30, 948.25, E890.9

17. Mr. John Detwiler had an esophagogastroduodenoscopy performed in the outpatient surgery unit. The appropriate code is:
    A. 43200
    B. 43226
    C. 43234
    D. 43235

18. The clinical resume final diagnostic statement reads: "Hiatal hernia, urinary tract infection, diabetes mellitus." The medication record indicates that the patient was administered Bactrim, Inderal, Diabinese, and Maalox. You would query the physician to add the following diagnosis to the statement:
    A. Chronic obstructive pulmonary disease
    B. Hypertension
    C. Sinus infection
    D. Headache

19. Mr. Steve Simpson had a left femoral herniorrhaphy for a recurrent reducible hernia. The appropriate code is:
    A. 49550
    B. 49553
    C. 49555
    D. 49557

20. Cindy Thompson was treated in the emergency room for lacerations of the left leg. Procedures performed include a layer closure of a 10 cm and 8 cm laceration. The appropriate code is:
    A. 12004
    B. 12035
    C. 12044
    D. 13121

21. A newborn delivered at Hospital A was immediately transferred to Hospital B to be monitored for drug intoxication (the mother is a cocaine abuser). The baby had no abnormal signs or symptoms and is discharged as a normal, healthy baby. The appropriate code for Hospital B to identify the principal diagnosis is:
    A. V29.8
    B. V30.00
    C. V30.1
    D. 760.75

22. The diagnosis on Mr. Smith's discharge summary reads: Congestive heart failure due to hypertensive heart disease with renal disease. The principal diagnosis is:
    A. 404.90
    B. 403.91
    C. 404.91
    D. 403.90

23. An inebriated 35-year-old male is admitted through the emergency room status post seizure with a 2-inch laceration of his temple. The laceration is sutured in the ER and the patient is admitted. Further tests reveal a lesion on the brain that is determined to be malignant. The principal diagnosis is:
    A. 191.9
    B. 780.3
    C. 873.49
    D. 305.0

24. A patient in ambulatory surgery unit undergoes bilateral needle biopsies of breasts. The appropriate code(s) is (are):
    A. 19100
    B. 19100, 19100
    C. 19101
    D. 19101, 19101

25. A patient being treated for a depressive disorder with Sinequan attends a party and drinks five mixed drinks. The patient becomes stuporous and is taken to the local ER for treatment. The appropriate codes are:
    A. 969.0, E854.0, 980.0, E860.0, 780.09
    B. 780.09, E860.9, E854.0
    C. 780.09, E950.3, E950.9
    D. 969.0, E854.0, E860.0, 780.09

26. A 55-year-old male is diagnosed with acute inferior wall myocardial infarction and arteriosclerotic heart disease. The following procedures are performed: coronary artery bypass graft × 2, internal mammary bypass graft × 1, intraoperative temporary pacemaker. The appropriate codes are:
    A. 410.41, 414.01, 36.12, 36.15, 39.61, 39.64
    B. 414.00, 410.40, 36.12, 36.15, 39.64
    C. 410.90, 414.00, 36.12, 36.15, 39.64
    D. 410.91, 414.01, 36.12, 36.15, 39.61, 39.64

27. Ms. Patsy King was admitted to an ambulatory surgery unit for an exploratory laparotomy and bilateral salpingo-oophorectomy. The appropriate code(s) is (are):
    A. 49000, 58940
    B. 58700
    C. 49000, 58720
    D. 58720

28. A 55-year-old patient has aortocoronary bypass of two coronary arteries with distal coronary endarterectomy, autologous blood transfusion. The appropriate codes are:
    A. 36.10, 38.1, 99.03
    B. 36.12, 39.61, 36.03, 99.02
    C. 39.59, 39.61, 99.0
    D. 36.12, 38.12, 99.0

29. Mrs. Barbara Collins is treated in the ambulatory surgery unit for removal of 25 skin tags of the right and left arms. The appropriate code(s) is (are):
    A. 11200
    B. 11200, 11201
    C. 11201
    D. 11400

30. David Jones is admitted for ectropion repair of the left lower lid with a full-thickness skin graft from the right upper lid. The procedure is performed in the outpatient surgery unit. The appropriate code(s) is (are):
    A. 67921, 67961
    B. 67961
    C. 67971
    D. 67973

Stop

80 Chapter 8

Answers and Explanations for Coding

1. **A** *Level:* Application   *Competency:* 1.2.7
   Source: Basic ICD-9-CM Coding Rules.

2. **C** *Level:* Application   *Competency:* 1.2.7
   Source: AHA Official Guideline 3.

3. **C** *Level:* Application   *Competency:* 1.2.7
   Source: AHA Official Guideline 7.

4. **C** *Level:* Application   *Competency:* 1.2.7
   Source: AHA Official Guideline 4.2.

5. **B** *Level:* Application   *Competency:* 1.2.7
   Source: AHA Official Guideline 2.13.

6. **C** *Level:* Application   *Competency:* 1.2.7
   Source: Basic ICD-9-CM Coding Rules.

7. **D** *Level:* Application   *Competency:* 1.2.7
   Source: AHA Official Guideline 2.16.

8. **C** *Level:* Application   *Competency:* 1.2.7
   Source: AHA Official Guideline 1.7.

9. **D** *Level:* Application   *Competency:* 1.2.7
   Source: AHA Official Guideline 2.13.

10. **D** *Level:* Application   *Competency:* 1.2.7
    Source: Basic ICD-9-CM Coding Rules.

11. **C** *Level:* Application   *Competency:* 1.1.29/1.1.31
    Source: AHA Official Guideline 1.7.

12. **D** *Level:* Application   *Competency:* 1.1.29/1.1.31
    Source: AHA Official Guideline 2.2.

13. **B** *Level:* Application   *Competency:* 1.1.29/1.1.31
    Source: Basic ICD-9-CM Coding Rules.

14. **C** *Level:* Application   *Competency:* 1.1.29/1.1.31
    Source: AHA Official Guideline 3.

15. **B** *Level:* Application *Competency:* 1.1.29/1.1.31
    Source: Basic ICD-9-CM Coding Rules.

16. **A** *Level:* Application *Competency:* 1.1.29/1.1.31
    Source: AHA Official Guideline 8.3.

17. **D** *Level:* Application *Competency:* 1.1.29/1.1.31
    Source: Basic ICD-9-CM Coding Rules.

18. **B** *Level:* Application *Competency:* 1.1.29/1.1.31
    Source: AHA Official Guideline 3.

19. **C** *Level:* Application *Competency:* 1.1.29/1.1.31
    Source: Basic ICD-9-CM Coding Rules.

20. **B** *Level:* Application *Competency:* 1.1.29/1.1.31
    Source: Basic ICD-9-CM Coding Rules.

21. **A** *Level:* Application *Competency:* 1.1.29/1.1.31
    Source: Basic ICD-9-CM Coding Rules.

22. **C** *Level:* Application *Competency:* 1.1.29/1.1.31
    Source: AHA Official Guideline 4.2.

23. **A** *Level:* Application *Competency:* 1.1.29/1.1.31
    Source: AHA Official Guideline 2.

24. **B** *Level:* Application *Competency:* 1.1.29/1.1.31
    Source: Basic ICD-9-CM Coding Rules.

25. **A** *Level:* Application *Competency:* 1.1.29/1.1.31
    Source: AHA Official Guideline 9.2.

26. **A** *Level:* Application *Competency:* 1.1.29/1.1.31
    Source: Basic ICD-9-CM Coding Rules.

27. **C** *Level:* Application *Competency:* 1.1.29/1.1.31
    Source: Basic ICD-9-CM Coding Rules.

28. **B** *Level:* Application *Competency:* 1.1.29/1.1.31
    Source: Basic ICD-9-CM Coding Rules.

29. **B** *Level:* Application   *Competency:* 1.1.29/1.1.31
    Source: Basic ICD-9-CM Coding Rules.

30. **C** *Level:* Application   *Competency:* 1.1.29/1.1.31
    Source: Basic ICD-9-CM Coding Rules.

Coding References for Further Study

American Hospital Association. *Official ICD-9-CM coding guidelines for coding and reporting.* Chicago: American Hospital Association.

American Hospital Association. *Coding Clinic for ICD-9-CM* (Quarterly publication of Central Office on ICD-9-CM).

Brown, F. (1994). *ICD-9-CM coding handbook* (1994 rev. ed.). American Hospital Association Publishing.

Huffman, E. K. (1994). *Health information management* (10th ed.). Berwyn, IL: Physicians' Record Company.

Nicholas, Toula (1995). *Basic ICD-9-CM coding handbook.* Chicago: American Health Information Management Association.

Nicholas, Toula (1995). *CPT/HCPCS basic coding handbook.* Chicago: American Health Information Management Association.

Chapter **9**

Legal Issues

Overview

This chapter deals with the legal issues surrounding the creation, maintenance, and safeguarding of the information in health records. A primary concern of health information practitioners is the release of information from the record to those who require that information. Such release must always protect the patient's right to privacy.

The particular competencies that are tested in this chapter are listed below, both for MRAs and MRTs.

MRA Competencies

1.1.14   Monitor accreditation/licensing survey results (i.e., Joint Commission, Medicare, etc.).
1.1.15   Monitor the release of information to ensure confidentiality of patient-related data.
1.1.17   Release patient-related data (i.e., reimbursement, research, legal, or patient-related purposes).
1.2.6   Compare data with other data sources or references to determine consistency.
3.1.9   Monitor policy or procedure compliance.

MRT Competencies

1.1.14   Monitor accreditation/licensing survey results (i.e., Joint Commission, Medicare, etc.).
1.1.15   Monitor the release of information to ensure confidentiality of patient-related data.
1.1.18   Release patient-related data (i.e., reimbursement, research, legal, or patient-related purposes).
1.2.6   Compare data with other data sources or references to determine consistency.
3.1.9   Monitor policy or procedure compliance.

Before you answer the questions, review your course material including all handouts, exercises, quizzes, and texts. Also review chapter 15 in *Health Information Management,* 10th edition (Huffman 1994). Answering the questions in this chapter will help the reader review knowledge and skills used in the legal aspects of health records.

Use one of the answer sheets provided for Chapter 9 to record your answers. Choose the one best answer for each item. Mark either A, B, C, or D for each question number.

Again, be sure to show any problem solving you did, either beside the question in the review book or on a separate sheet of paper. This will help you retrace your steps and let you determine whether you made a careless error in math or reading. If you continue to make many of these kinds of errors, refer to Chapter 1 again, which reviews test-taking strategies. Also note if you had to guess at the answer by placing a question mark or other symbol beside the question. Guessing is an important clue that you may need more information about this topic.

After you answer the questions, check your choices against the answers and explanations provided. Use the number of questions that you answered correctly to calculate your score using the grid on the answer sheet. Again indicate those materials that you would like to review further before the national exam.

Place the score for this chapter on the separate grid that is provided. The grid will allow you to determine your overall score when you have completed all the tests. You will want to do further review in those areas where you record the lowest scores. References for study are provided at the end of the chapter.

Test Items

Legal Questions

Number of Items: 20
MRA Time Allowed: 18 minutes
MRT Time Allowed: 19 minutes

Start

1. An insurance company has requested copies of a patient's records. The patient has been diagnosed as having AIDS. The hospital's policy for release of information in this instance should ensure that the:
   A. Record is sent by certified mail
   B. Physician gives consent for a copy of the record to be released
   C. Patient has signed a consent specifically authorizing release of this diagnosis
   D. HIM director discusses this with the patient prior to sending copies

2. A properly completed and signed authorization is required for release of all health information except when a(n):
   A. Patient requests information sent to another physician
   B. Patient presents for treatment in the emergency room
   C. Insurance company requests copies of the patient's last hospitalization
   D. Patient's spouse requests copies sent to another physician

3. A good example of respondeat superior is:
   A. The judge recognized the truthful existence (evidence) of certain facts
   B. Mary gives money to Joan to be held in trust
   C. A person gives testimony that no one else can give
   D. The hospital is held responsible for a nurse's medication error

4. As director of Health Information Management (HIM) you have been subpoenaed to court. You are qualified to testify in response to a subpoena duces tecum that the record is:
   A. Maintained in the hospital's regular order of business
   B. Accurate and complete
   C. Compiled by competent health care providers whose authentications are so noted
   D. A confidential document with physician/patient statutory privileges

5. A statute of limitations law is important in that it:
   A. Defines an important limitation upon liability of hospitals
   B. Sets a minimum amount of time after an event occurs for a suit to be taken to court
   C. Sets a time period for releasing records to an attorney
   D. Is a formal obligation to do a certain act that is then recorded in court

6. In the absence of state law, medical records should be maintained in those facilities that treat Medicare/Medicaid adult patients for:
   A. A minimum of 10 years
   B. 5 years from date of discharge
   C. 25 years
   D. 15 years

7. A subpoena should be refused in all of the following cases except when:
   A. The name of the court is not present on the subpoena
   B. The date, time, and place of appearance is not stated on the subpoena
   C. The signature of the patient is not present on the subpoena
   D. The signature of the official empowered to issue the subpoena is not present on the subpoena

8. Refusing to honor a subpoena may result in:
   A. Arrest
   B. Being considered in contempt of court
   C. Judicial fines being imposed
   D. Another subpoena being issued

9. The doctrine of res ipsa loquitur can be illustrated in which of the following cases:
   A. A surgeon nicks a ureter during tubal ligation
   B. A surgeon performs an appendectomy on a patient found after surgery to have a normal appendix
   C. A nurse neglects to give postoperative pain medication as ordered
   D. A surgeon leaves a surgical instrument in the body of a patient unintentionally

10. You are the supervisor of the Release of Information section of the HIM department in a government-owned hospital. The rules of the department outline access to the record conforming to the Uniform Healthcare Information Act, which grants the patient the right to inspect, copy, and amend the medical record. A nursing student from the local community college submits a request to view a record of a patient in her care. Your response would be to:
    A. Deny access
    B. Obtain consent of the attending physician
    C. Obtain consent of the patient
    D. Allow viewing of the record if you are present and the student has the instructor's approval

11. A patient has a primary diagnosis of cocaine abuse and dependence. The following information items may be released without the patient's consent:
    A. Admission and discharge dates only
    B. No information, including the fact that he was treated at the facility
    C. The patient's name only
    D. The patient's name, address, sex, age, and attending physician

12. A manager at the Sunnyside Car Wash calls the HIM department to say that one of his employees is in the hospital. Since his company carries its own medical insurance for all employees, the company is the identified guarantor for the employee's hospital bill. The manager asks that you send him a resume upon discharge of the patient. You may send him the resume:
    A. If the attending physician agrees
    B. If the patient signs a written authorization
    C. If the administrator approves the request
    D. Because his company is paying the hospital bill

13. Larry Smith contacted the HIM department stating that he had recently received the requested copies of his medical records to take to an out-of-state physician he is consulting. He also stated there is an error in the past medical history of his record. He wants the information corrected. As director of the HIM department your course of action would be to:
    A. Draw a line through the incorrect information and write in the corrected statement
    B. Contact the attending physician and request that he/she correct the information
    C. Inform the patient that there is no recourse for him to have this information corrected
    D. Inform the patient that he can request that an amendment be made to the original entry by insertion of an additional document with the corrected information

14. Getwell Hospital's HIM department processes over 350 requests for information per month. Departmental policy and compliance with federal guidelines requires that all information released from the department be stamped with a statement that documents:
    A. That the release was recorded in the Release of Information Log Book
    B. A notice that the information has been recorded on the activity sheet in the patient's record
    C. A Redisclosure Statement to warn against unauthorized release to another institution
    D. An itemization of the charges for the release of this patient's records

15. An agent of the IRS wants to look at the names and addresses of the patients seen by a particular physician. The HIM director should:
    A. Call the hospital attorney
    B. Call the security officer
    C. Give the agent the information requested
    D. Refuse to provide the information

16. As director of Health Information Services, you have received a letter from a former patient stating that she has moved. She requests that a copy of her medical record be mailed to her new physician and provides his name and address. You should:
    A. Mail the record to the doctor as no further authorization is necessary
    B. Refer the question to the hospital's attorney
    C. Send the woman the proper hospital authorization form
    D. Wait for the woman's new doctor to request the record

17. Hospital policy allows release of information over the telephone after confirming the identity of the caller. The supervisor of the release of information section observes one of the employees receiving a non-urgent telephone request for information on a patient. Laying the phone down, the clerk checks the Master Patient Index. The entry for the patient indicates "NO INFORMATION" stamped in big red letters. The clerk returns to the phone and politely tells the party there is no information to release. The supervisor requests a meeting with the employee to instruct the employee in the proper procedure for this type of situation. The clerk is reminded to ask the requestor the reason the information is needed, take the name and phone number of the caller, and:
    A. Tell the caller, "Please call back in 5 minutes and I'll have the information for you"
    B. Indicate that she will return the call, but after checking the information, not return the call
    C. Indicate that she will return the call, and after checking the information, she tells the requesting party there is no information to release.
    D. Refer the call to the supervisor

18. An employer telephones the HIM department and requests the medical records of an employee, to be used to verify hospitalization. The release of information clerk efficiently sends a copy of the full record. As a result of the information contained in the record, the employee is fired. The former patient, seeking restitution, sues the hospital under the doctrine of:
    A. Official public records rule
    B. Res gestae
    C. Respondeat superior
    D. Workers' compensation

19. The Cornerstone Foundation provides a home for children of families who cannot care for them. A child from this home comes to your hospital for a scheduled umbilical hernia repair. Mr. Adams, the superintendent of Cornerstone, is with the child and states that he will sign the authorization for hospital care and for surgery. Before the operation can proceed, you need to:
    A. Get authorization from the child's parents
    B. Obtain a court order
    C. Get authorization from a representative of the State Department of Health
    D. Determine who has legal custody of the child

20. Larry Jones, age 17, was abandoned at the age of 4 and reared by foster parents. At age 16 he left his foster parents and started making his own living. He was recently married to Debbie, who is 22. Larry now needs to have an arthroscopy with a medial meniscectomy. Consent for this surgery should be given by:
    A. Larry
    B. Larry's wife, Debbie
    C. Larry's foster parents
    D. Both Larry and Debbie

Stop

Answers and Explanations for Legal Issues

1. **C** *Level:* Application *Competency:* 1.1.15
   Source: Huffman, (1994), pages 587–588.

2. **B** *Level:* Knowledge *Competency:* 1.1.17/1.1.18
   Source: Huffman (1994), pages 584–586.

3. **D** *Level:* Application *Competency:* 1.1.15
   Source: Roach (1994), page 269.

4. **A** *Level:* Knowledge *Competency:* 1.1.17/1.1.18
   Source: Huffman (1994), pages 592–602.

5. **A** *Level:* Knowledge *Competency:* 1.1.15
   Rationale: Statutes of limitation are determined by each state. This is the period of time after discovery of an event in which legal action can be initiated. It may be years before the case goes to court.
   Source: Huffman (1990), page 307.

6. **A** *Level:* Knowledge *Competency:* 1.1.14
   Source: Huffman (1994), pages 305–307.

7. **C** *Level:* Knowledge *Competency:* 1.1.15
   Source: Huffman (1994), pages 593–594.

8. **B** *Level:* Knowledge *Competency:* 1.1.15
   Source: Huffman (1994), pages 593–594.

9. **D** *Level:* Application *Competency:* 1.2.6
   Rationale: Res ipsa loquitur means "the thing stands for itself." In this case, an expert witness is not needed to testify that instruments are not normally left inside the patient.
   Source: Roach (1994), page 674.

10. **D** *Level:* Application *Competency:* 1.1.17/1.1.18
    Source: Huffman (1994), pages 584–585.

11. **B** *Level:* Knowledge *Competency:* 1.1.17/1.1.18
    Source: Huffman (1994), pages 581–582.

12. **B** *Level:* Application   *Competency:* 1.1.17/1.1.18
    Source: Huffman (1994), pages 584–592.

13. **D** *Level:* Application   *Competency:* 1.1.17/1.1.18
    Source: Huffman (1994), pages 575–576.

14. **C** *Level:* Knowledge   *Competency:* 1.1.17/1.1.18
    Source: Huffman (1994), page 586.

15. **D** *Level:* Application   *Competency:* 1.1.17/1.1.18
    Source: Huffman (1994), pages 576–579.

16. **A** *Level:* Application   *Competency:* 1.1.17/1.1.18
    Rationale: To have a letter from the woman indicating her wishes about her medical record information is better than having a particular hospital authorization completed and signed.

17. **C** *Level:* Problem solving   *Competency:* 1.1.15
    Rationale: Returning a telephone call is one way to confirm the identity of the caller.

18. **C** *Level:* Application   *Competency:* 3.1.9
    Rationale: The doctrine of respondeat superior holds the organization responsible for an employee's actions when they are following the policy of the organization. What we do not know is whether there was an established policy that would have prohibited the employee's behavior. If there is and the employee had been properly instructed in the procedure for following the policy, the hospital would have a legal defense in this case. However, if there was no policy or the employee was not properly trained in the procedures, the hospital is legally responsible for the employee's actions.

19. **D** *Level:* Application   *Competency:* 3.1.9
    Rationale: The legal status of this child regarding custody would have to be determined before any decision about authorizing surgery can be made.

20. **A** *Level:* Application   *Competency:* 1.1.17/1.1.18

    Rationale: In most states, a minor who becomes financially independent is known as an "emancipated minor" and has the same right to consent to medical care as any adult. There is no need for the spouse to consent for this type of procedure, as would be desirable in procedures that affect the reproductive capacity of an individual.

Legal References for Further Study

Cowdrey, M. (1990). *Basic law for the allied health professions.* Monterey, CA: Wadsworth, Inc.

Huffman, E. K. (1994). *Health information management* (10th ed.). Berwyn, IL: Physicians' Record Company.

Miller, *Problems in health law* (6th ed.). Gaithersburg, MA: Aspen Publishers, Inc.

Roach, William H., Jr. (1994). *Medical records and the law* (2nd ed.). Gaithersburg, MA: Aspen Publishers, Inc.

Chapter 10

Management

Overview

This chapter deals with the management of operations within a Health Information Management (HIM) department. Management involves efficiently and effectively using internal and external resources to meet objectives. The four functions of management, as defined by Huffman (1994), are planning, organizing, directing, and controlling. Planning includes the development of specific objectives. Meeting these objectives requires organization of tasks and the people necessary to complete those tasks. Job simplification and good work flow are necessary. Controls must be set in place to ensure that the objectives are, in fact, accomplished.

Management skills are crucial for MRAs but are also important for MRTs as both levels of health information practitioners are often given responsibility for departments or units within a department.

The particular competencies that are tested in this chapter are listed below, both for MRAs and MRTs.

MRA Competencies

1.1.25 Confer with peers, providers, or users of departmental or institutional services.
2.1.1 Develop departmental plans, goals, and objectives for areas under your span of control.
2.1.5 Develop or revise job descriptions.

2.1.14   Design departmental operational systems for information retention and retrieval (i.e, filing systems, filing equipment, retention policies/procedures, etc.).
2.2.6   Determine personnel needs for staffing current or new systems.
2.2.8   Determine space requirements for current or new systems.
3.1.2   Train personnel.
3.1.3   Inform organization staff of plan(s).
3.1.4   Implement new or revised policies and procedures.
3.1.7   Monitor adherence to budget (i.e., determine budget variance, etc.).
3.1.12   Design employee staffing schedules.
3.1.15   Conduct educational programs for departmental or nondepartmental staff.
4.1.2   Determine variation(s) from established objective or standards of performance.
4.1.3   Recommend changes or improvement(s) in systems.

MRT Competencies

1.1.26   Confer with peers, providers, or users of departmental or institutional services.
2.1.1   Develop departmental plans, goals, and objectives for areas under your span of control.
2.1.4   Develop or revise job descriptions.
2.1.5   Design transition plans for implementation of new or revised systems.
2.2.1   Determine personnel needs for staffing current or new systems.
2.2.3   Determine space requirements for current or new systems.
3.1.2   Train personnel.
3.1.3   Inform organization staff of plan(s).
3.1.4   Implement new or revised policies and procedures.
3.1.7   Monitor adherence to budget (i.e., determine budget variance, etc.).
3.1.12   Design employee staffing schedules.
3.1.15   Conduct educational programs for departmental or nondepartmental staff.
4.1.2   Determine variation(s) from established objective or standards of performance.
4.1.3   Recommend changes or improvement(s) in systems.

Before you answer the questions, review your course material including all handouts, exercises, quizzes, and texts. Also review chapter 17 in *Health Information Management,* 10th edition (Huffman 1994). Answering the questions in this chapter will help the reader review knowledge and skills used in the management of a health information department or supervision of a function within the department.

Use one of the answer sheets provided for Chapter 10 to record your answers. Choose the one best answer for each item. Mark either A, B, C, or D for each question number.

Again, be sure to show any problem solving you did, either beside the question in the review book or on a separate sheet of paper. This will help you retrace your steps and let you determine whether you made a careless error in math or reading. If you continue to make many of these kinds of errors, refer to Chapter 1 again, which reviews test-taking strategies. Also note if you had to guess at the answer by placing a question mark or other symbol beside the question. Guessing is an important clue that you may need more information about this topic.

After you answer the questions, check your choices against the answers and explanations provided. Use the number of questions that you answered correctly to calculate your score using the grid on the answer sheet. Again indicate those materials that you would like to review further before the national exam.

Place the score for this chapter on the separate grid that is provided. The grid will allow you to determine your overall score when you have completed all the tests. You will want to do further review in those areas where you record the lowest scores. References for study are provided at the end of the chapter.

Test Items

Management Questions

Number of Items: 25
MRA Time Allowed: 24 minutes
MRT Time Allowed: 25 minutes

Start

1. Each month, the Health Information Management department director reviews the departmental budget report and analyzes the variances between the proposed and the actual expenditures. The management process that <u>underlies</u> this activity is:

    A. Planning
    B. Organizing
    C. Directing
    D. Controlling

2. The department's first quarter budget analysis shows that while the expected cost of operations was $227,200, the actual cost of operations was $239,875. The budget variance is:

    A. 0.5%
    B. 5.3%
    C. 5.6%
    D. 7.2%

3. The statement "Using ICD-9-CM, assign code numbers to diagnoses listed on 50 patient records each day with 98% accuracy" is an example of a(n)

    A. Strategic plan
    B. Objective
    C. Mission statement
    D. Policy

4. The following budget information is being used to evaluate the performance of the HIM department manager.

	1994	
	Actual	**Budgeted**
Number of Discharges	100,000	120,000
Variable Costs	$1,200,000	$1,320,000
Fixed Costs	600,000	600,000
Total Costs	$1,800,000	$1,920,000

The manager, of course, is not responsible for the decreased volume of discharges. Variance analysis of the information reveals:

A. The actual cost per discharge was the same as that budgeted
B. The actual cost per discharge decreased proportionate to the decrease in variable costs
C. The actual variable cost per discharge increased even though the actual dollar amount shows a favorable variance
D. A favorable variance in variable costs and no further analysis will be done

5. A coder within the HIM department is expected to accurately code 10 records per hour. The hospital has 25,000 annual discharges. Assume that an employee works 2080 hours per year. Nonproductive time accounts for 10% of the total hours worked per year. The number of full-time employees needed to perform the coding function is:

A. 1.20
B. 1.28
C. 2.0
D. 1.34

6. The HIM department is open from 6:00 A.M. to 11:00 P.M., 7 days a week. Two employees are required on duty at all times. The minimum number of employees required for adequate coverage is:

A. 2.98
B. 4.25
C. 5.95
D. 8.50

7. When comparing department performance against standards that have been established, the HIM director is performing the function of:
   A. Planning
   B. Organizing
   C. Directing
   D. Controlling

8. As an HIM director, you pay a coder $11 per hour. This is a full-time position at 2080 hours per year. The cost for fringe benefits for a full time employee is 24% of the employee's salary. The annual gross cost for this employee is:
   A. $22,880
   B. $24,371
   C. $26,822
   D. $28,371

9. For a 2-week period, the HIM department had 1200 worked hours and 1280 total (or paid) hours on its payroll report. During this same 2 weeks, there were 375 discharges. The department's standard for staffing is 3.3 worked hours per discharge. The number of worked hours per discharge was:
   A. 3.0
   B. 3.2
   C. 3.4
   D. 3.8

10. When the HIM director prepares the annual budget, the function being performed is:
    A. Planning
    B. Organizing
    C. Directing
    D. Controlling

11. The director has decided that the assistant director of record processing will be promoted to associate director of the department. A coder will assume the duties of supervising the record processing section. The director is performing the management function of:
    A. Planning
    B. Organizing
    C. Directing
    D. Controlling

12. The health information manager exercises staff authority in the hospital when he/she:
    A. Abstracts a medical record
    B. Advises on a file system for the radiology department
    C. Teaches a file clerk a procedure
    D. Writes a procedure for the correct filing of records

13. A supervisor who spends time on tasks that others could perform satisfactorily has the fault of:
    A. Inefficient planning
    B. Unnecessary changes
    C. Failure to delegate
    D. Lack of proper control of employees

14. You are supervising the coding section of a large hospital. You are concerned that the poor work flow is contributing to lost time for these employees. A simple tool that facilitates checking that furniture and equipment are placed effectively in a health information department layout is:
    A. Gantt chart
    B. Managerial grid
    C. Movement diagram
    D. PERT network

15. The human resource department at your facility is revising the wage and salary program. The documents that could be requested from you as director of HIM to facilitate the revisions are:
    A. Job descriptions
    B. Job procedures
    C. Policies
    D. Performance appraisals

16. As manager of the HIM department you have determined that you need to hire two additional employees in the filing and retrieval area. In conjunction with the human resource department of your facility you begin the process of job analysis. The first step would be for you to:
    A. Assess how and when job candidates should be evaluated
    B. Collect data based on criteria
    C. Decide what kinds of data to collect
    D. Write the job description

17. Sally Givens is supervisor of the Release of Information section in the HIM department. The authority that she exerts when she directs the employees in this section is referred to as:
    A. Functional
    B. Line
    C. Coercive
    D. Staff

18. The use of a project management tool would be ideal for:
    A. Converting files to a new system over a weekend
    B. Gathering budget data
    C. Monitoring productivity of new employees
    D. Using new transcription equipment for one month trial period

19. A chart of organization is important because it:
    A. Demonstrates relationships between departments and points out shortcomings
    B. Ensures good organization
    C. Takes the place of policy manuals and procedures
    D. Identifies informal relationships and power sources

20. The health information manager discussed laser disk technology with the vice president for the health information and data information departments. The vice president was enthusiastic and suggested a work group be formed by these two departments to discuss the new technology and develop recommendations for the facility. This work group is an example of:
    A. Informal coordinating mechanism
    B. Standing committee with line authority
    C. Formal coordinating mechanism
    D. Temporary committee with line authority

21. "The institution will maintain security measures and provide the staff and facilities necessary to safeguard the property and personal safety of employees, patients, and the public" is an example of a:
    A. Method
    B. Policy
    C. Procedure
    D. Rule

Use the following information to answer questions 22 and 23.

> The manager and assistant manager of a HIM department are planning for the number of employees needed for the coming years as they establish goals. They review several articles in current health care publications that describe new regulations that could impact the amount of time an abstractor spends on each patient record. Other articles tell of a breakthrough in computer technology that could increase the likelihood of implementing a true computer-based patient record.

22. The activities of the manager and assistant manager in reviewing these articles can be described as the planning subfunction of:
    A. Assessing the external environment
    B. Assessing the internal environment
    C. Defining the course of action to achieve an outcome
    D. Setting objectives for the coming year

23. The managers choose to ignore the information in the articles. Six months after submitting their plan for the coming year they learn that they need one additional employee to meet the new abstracting requirements. This is an example of:
    A. Anticipating change and responding to new requirements
    B. Crisis management in the planning function
    C. Developing objectives as part of decision-making activities
    D. Wise operational planning and organizing

24. The HIM manager is planning for completion of the steps needed to prepare the budget for the next year. A good tool for developing a time line and tracking progress against this time line is a:
    A. Flowchart
    B. Flow process chart
    C. GANTT chart
    D. PERT chart

25. The admissions office manager in an acute-care facility asks the HIM manager to prepare and present an in-service program that will help the admitting clerks understand their role in the interaction between the departments, especially with documentation on the face sheet. An outcome for this in-service program relating to the admitting diagnoses would best state that after the program the admitting clerks will:
   A. Assign the patient to the appropriate floor based on the admitting diagnosis 95% of the time
   B. Correctly code the admitting diagnosis 95% of the time
   C. Correctly pronounce an appropriate admitting diagnosis 95% of the time
   D. Enter the appropriate admitting diagnosis on the inpatient face sheet 95% of the time

Stop

Answers and Explanations for Management

1. **D** *Level:* Application *Competency:* 4.1.2/4.1.1
   Source: Huffman (1994), pages 701–702.

2. **B** *Level:* Problem solving *Competency:* 3.1.7
   Rationale: Dollar amount of variance = $239,875 − $227,200 = $12,675/$227,200 = 5.6

3. **B** *Level:* Application *Competency:* 2.1.1
   Source: Huffman (1994), page 652.

4. **C** *Level:* Problem solving *Competency:* 3.1.7
   Rationale: Variable cost divided by the number of units (discharges) shows the actual variable cost to be $12 per discharge ($1,200,000/100,000) and the budgeted variable cost is $11 per discharge ($1,320,000/120,000).

5. **D** *Level:* Problem solving *Competency:* 2.2.6/2.2.1
   Rationale: $2500/2080 − (2080 \times .10) = 1.34$

6. **C** *Level:* Problem solving *Competency:* 2.2.6/2.2.1
   Rationale: 6 A.M. − 11 P.M. = 17 hours. $17 \times 2 = 34 \times 7 = 238/40 = 5.95$.

7. **D** *Level:* Application *Competency:* 4.1.2/4.1.1
   Source: Huffman (1994), page 667.

8. **D** *Level:* Problem solving *Competency:* 2.2.6/2.2.1
   Rationale: $2080 \times 11 \times 1.24 = \$28,371$

9. **B** *Level:* Problem solving *Competency:* 2.2.6/2.2.1
   Rationale: $1200/375 = 3.2$

10. **A** *Level:* Application *Competency:* 2.1.1
    Source: Huffman (1994), pages 655–664.

11. **B** *Level:* Application *Competency:* 4.1.3/4.1.2
    Source: Huffman (1994), page 671.

12. **B** *Level:* Application *Competency:* 1.1.25/1.1.26

   Rationale: Line positions have direct responsibility for accomplishing objectives. The HIM director has this type of position within the department. However, when assisting or advising people in the organization outside the HIM department, the HIM manager is performing a staff function. Legal counsel and human resources professionals are often referred to as having staff positions within the organization; however, these individuals often have line responsibility within their own departments or areas.

   Source: Huffman (1994), pages 673–675.

13. **C** *Level:* Application *Competency:* 3.1.2
   Source: Huffman (1994), pages 675–676.

14. **C** *Level:* Application *Competency:* 2.2.8/2.2.3
   Source: Huffman (1994), pages 680–683.

15. **A** *Level:* Application *Competency:* 2.1.5/2.1.4
   Source: Huffman (1994), pages 724–725.

16. **C** *Level:* Application *Competency:* 2.2.6/2.2.1
   Source: Huffman (1994), pages 723–725.

17. **B** *Level:* Application *Competency:* 3.1.3
   Source: Huffman (1994), pages 673–675.

18. **A** *Level:* Application *Competency:* 2.1.14
   Source: Huffman (1994), pages 667–669.

19. **A** *Level:* Knowledge *Competency:* 2.1.1
   Source: Huffman (1994), pages 676–678.

20. **C** *Level:* Application *Competency:* 2.1.1
   Source: Huffman (1994), pages 672–673.

21. **C** *Level:* Application *Competency:* 3.1.4
   Source: Huffman (1994), page 664.

22. **A** *Level:* Application *Competency:* 4.1.3/4.1.2
   Source: Huffman (1994), page 652.

23. **B** *Level:* Application *Competency:* 4.1.3/4.1.2
    Source: Huffman (1994), pages 650–651.

24. **C** *Level:* Application *Competency:* 3.1.12
    Source: Huffman (1994), pages 667–668.

25. **D** *Level:* Application *Competency:* 3.1.15
    Source: Huffman (1994), page 648.

Management References for Further Study

Huffman, E. K. (1994). *Health information management* (10th ed.). Berwyn, IL: Physicians' Record Company.

Kallaus, N. F. & Keeling, B. L. (1991). *Administrative office management* (10th ed.). Cincinnati, OH: South-Western Publishing Co.

Longest, B. (1990). *Management practices for the health professional.* Norwalk, CT: Appleton & Lange.

Rakich, J. S., Longest, B. B., & Darr, K. (1992). *Managing health services organizations* (3rd ed.). Baltimore, MD: Health Professions Press.

Chapter 11

Human Resource Management

Overview

This chapter deals with the human resource aspects of Health Information Management (HIM). This includes the management and supervision of people. Both MRA and MRT students must know how to get work accomplished. Motivation of employees is important, as well as clear communications. No matter how good your objectives are, you cannot accomplish these objectives without the help of employees in the unit or department.

The competencies that are tested in this chapter, for both MRAs and MRTs, are listed below.

MRA Competencies

- 1.1.25 Confer with peers, providers, or users of departmental or institutional services.
- 2.2.6 Determine personnel needs for staffing current or new systems.
- 3.1.1 Select personnel.
- 3.1.3 Inform organization staff of plan(s).
- 3.1.4 Implement new or revised policies and procedures.
- 3.1.10 Counsel or discipline employees.
- 4.1.3 Recommend changes or improvement(s) in systems.
- 4.1.4 Evaluate employee performance.

MRT Competencies

- 1.1.26 Confer with peers, providers, or users of departmental or institutional services.

2.2.1   Determine personnel needs for staffing current or new systems.
3.1.1   Select personnel.
3.1.3   Inform organization staff of plan(s).
3.1.4   Implement new or revised policies and procedures.
3.1.10 Counsel or discipline employees.
4.1.2   Recommend changes or improvement(s) in systems.
4.1.3   Evaluate employee performance.

Before you answer the questions, review your course material including all handouts, exercises, quizzes, and texts. Also review chapter 18 in *Health Information Management,* 10th edition (Huffman 1994). Answering the questions in this chapter will help the reader review knowledge and skills used in the management and supervision of people in a health information department or a function within the department.

Use one of the answer sheets provided for Chapter 11 to record your answers. Choose the one best answer for each item. Mark either A, B, C, or D for each question number.

Again, be sure to show any problem solving you did, either beside the question in the review book or on a separate sheet of paper. This will help you retrace your steps and let you determine whether you made a careless error in math or reading. If you continue to make many of these kinds of errors, refer to Chapter 1 again, which reviews test-taking strategies. Also note if you had to guess at the answer by placing a question mark or other symbol beside the question. Guessing is an important clue that you may need more information about this topic.

After you answer the questions, check your choices against the answers and explanations provided. Use the number of questions that you answered correctly to calculate your score using the grid on the answer sheet. Again indicate those materials that you would like to review further before the national exam.

Place the score for this chapter on the separate grid that is provided. The grid will allow you to determine your overall score when you have completed all the tests. You will want to do further review in those areas where you record the lowest scores. References for study are provided at the end of the chapter.

Before you answer the questions, review your course material and chapter 18 in Huffman (1994). Answering the questions that follow will help you determine if further review is needed.

Test Items

Human Resource Management Questions

Number of Items: 20
MRA Time Allowed: 18 minutes
MRT Time Allowed: 19 minutes

Start

1. Utilization management is a part of the HIM department. The HIM director is informed by the director of nursing that a utilization review coordinator has breached confidential information. The HIM director's first course of action should be to:
   A. Immediately terminate the employee
   B. Document the problem for future reference
   C. Privately counsel the employee
   D. Discuss the consequences of breach of confidentiality at the next departmental meeting

2. A question that would be helpful in opening up the issue of an employee's unsatisfactory performance is:
   A. "Are you aware of your error rate versus the departmental error rate?"
   B. "Do you realize you are a problem for me because you are never on time?"
   C. "Are you aware that you are the slowest employee in the department?"
   D. "Can you explain why you are so slow and ignorant?"

3. As manager of the HIM department you want to implement a system where the coders' salary structure is based on actual work produced. This type of pay system is referred to as:
   A. Hourly
   B. Incentive
   C. Merit
   D. Productive

4. When an employee disagrees with elements of the performance appraisal and offers specific information to refute the findings, you should:
   A. Ask the employee to leave
   B. Indicate your willingness to reexamine your data
   C. Request that the employee meet with you and the human resource director to discuss the problem
   D. Tell the employee to document his/her disagreement and you will file it in his/her personnel file

5. The HIM director is interviewing candidates for the position of file clerk supervisor. Responsibilities for this position include daily scheduling and control of file room activities, supervision and evaluation of file room personnel, maintenance of file room procedures, and working with hospital personnel in solving problems. The least appropriate qualification that an applicant could possess is:
   A. Good interpersonal skills
   B. Supervisory experience
   C. Analytical ability for problem solving
   D. Excellent oral and written communication skills

6. As supervisor of the transcription section you want to get some information to the transcriptionists about possible changes in the organizational structure without using formal communication. The method of communication you could use is the:
   A. Employee handbook
   B. Grapevine
   C. House newsletter
   D. Notice with their paycheck

7. The following situations have all occurred during a day you experience as manager of the HIM department. An example of informal communication channels is:
   A. An employee asks you for a week of vacation
   B. You provide in-service training for the department employees
   C. You conduct a departmental meeting
   D. The director of radiology asks your advice about selecting dictation equipment

Use the following information to answer questions 8 through 11:

Mildred Benson has been employed as a coder in the Health Information Management department for 5 years. She is considered the top coder as her work is very accurate and she maintains a high productivity rate. She is well liked by all of the employees. Mildred is always friendly, willing to help others, and makes an effort to ensure that everything is running smoothly.

It has become apparent lately that Mildred is not her usual self. During the past 2 months her productivity has dropped and her error rate has increased. She appears withdrawn and preoccupied with her own thoughts. She does not converse much with others and on several occasions has become irritated and ill-tempered. A tardiness pattern is also developing.

8. The most appropriate action for the supervisor to take at this time is to:
   A. Do nothing because of the fear of interfering with Mildred's personal life
   B. Ask the other employees if they know what is wrong
   C. Call Mildred in for a counseling session to determine causes and possible remedies
   D. Document Mildred's tardiness and dock her pay for the accumulated absence of time for the pay period

9. If the other employees complain to the supervisor she should:
   A. Ask one of them to try to find out what is wrong
   B. Assure them she is aware of the situation and that efforts are under way to remedy the problems
   C. Share with them any additional information she may have concerning the situation and discuss actions being taken
   D. Tell the others they should mind their own business and let the supervisor handle things

10. If the supervisor decides to talk with Mildred about the situation at this point, the supervisor should:
    A. Talk informally with Mildred about the situation, try to work out some solutions together, and write notes for Mildred's departmental file
    B. Talk to Mildred about the situation, explain to her that this is a formal counseling session and document it as such in her personnel file

C. Suspend Mildred temporarily without pay
D. Terminate Mildred because of tardiness, drop in productivity, and increased error rate

11. If Mildred came to the supervisor on her own initiative to discuss the situation, the supervisor should most appropriately:
    A. Listen openly and willingly to what Mildred has to say, then make a referral to EAP (employee assistance program) if needed
    B. Explain to Mildred that if she is here to discuss personal problems, then this is not the supervisor's responsibility as personal issues should be left at home
    C. Explain to Mildred that she will listen to her side of the story but that she also has questions for her
    D. Use this as an opportunity to inform Mildred of her unacceptable behavior and actions and then document this as a formal counseling session

12. A transcriptionist is editing out terms and phrases in dictation. A physician discusses changes in a discharge summary with the transcription supervisor and states that reports have shown edits in the past but he had not mentioned it to the supervisor. Based on the information above, the appropriate action for the supervisor would be to review a sample of the employee's work and:
    A. Issue an oral reprimand to the employee
    B. Take no action at this point, since it is not a major problem
    C. Issue an oral reprimand with a written record placed in the employee's personnel file
    D. Informally counsel the employee at the employee's workstation

13. The director of the HIM department has contacted you concerning questions he has about the performance evaluations for employees in the filing area. The evaluations conducted indicate marginal performance by some of the employees. As the supervisor, the first step to take in assessing the problem is to review the:
    A. Salary scale for the filing area
    B. Employee's understanding of expectations
    C. Expectations of the department director
    D. Work standards and job descriptions

14. Employee performance appraisals may be used for all of the following purposes except to:
    A. Uncover exceptional skills among employees
    B. Study and analyze jobs held by employees
    C. Aid in settling disputes in arbitration cases
    D. Identify prospective movement by employees within the organization

Use the following information to answer questions 15 and 16:

Yearly performance appraisals are scheduled to begin in 2 months for the file clerks. In planning for these appraisals, the assistant director of the HIM department reviewed the job descriptions for these positions. The reviews revealed the need for revisions since the file clerks are now using an automated record-tracking system. These job descriptions were last reviewed 2 years ago.

15. The best first step the assistant director can take is to:
    A. Initiate revision of job specifications based on the evaluation of a file clerk's performance
    B. Undertake a job analysis using observation, interviewing, daily time logs, and other techniques
    C. Revise the job to match the job description
    D. Conduct the performance appraisals as things are now

16. The computer skills needed for the change to automation will upgrade the job specifications; this will also:
    A. Standardize the job description of the file clerk supervisor
    B. Standardize the organizational chart of the department
    C. Enhance the opportunity for raising the file clerk's wage scale
    D. Document compliance with the accrediting mandates for the facility

17. The major part of the performance appraisal feedback interview should be spent discussing:
    A. Past accomplishments
    B. Weaknesses of the employee
    C. Strengths of the employee
    D. Future goals and improvements

18. When a union is being considered by employees, an employer can:
    A. Ask employees for information about organizing activities
    B. Attend union meetings or try to find out who is participating
    C. Tell employees of the disadvantages of belonging to a union
    D. Visit employees at home to urge them to oppose the union
19. The first step in applying discipline of an employee for a first offense is:
    A. Termination
    B. Suspension
    C. Oral reprimand
    D. Written warning
20. The most important task in handling an employee grievance is:
    A. Making a quick decision
    B. Getting information about the grievance
    C. Writing down a description of the grievance
    D. Notifying the personnel department about the grievance

Stop

Answers and Explanations for Human Resource Management

1. **C** *Level:* Application *Competency:* 3.1.10
   Source: Huffman (1994), pages 732–733.

2. **A** *Level:* Application *Competency:* 4.1.4/4.1.3
   Source: Huffman (1994), pages 739–743.

3. **B** *Level:* Knowledge *Competency:* 4.1.3/4.1.2
   Source: Huffman (1994), pages 739–743.

4. **B** *Level:* Application *Competency:* 4.1.4/4.1.3
   Source: Huffman (1994), pages 739–743.

5. **D** *Level:* Application *Competency:* 3.1.1
   Source: Huffman (1994), pages 725–729.

6. **B** *Level:* Knowledge *Competency:* 3.1.3
   Source: Huffman (1994), pages 714–719.

7. **A** *Level:* Application *Competency:* 2.2.6/2.2.1
   Source: Huffman (1994), pages 714–719.

8. **C** *Level:* Application *Competency:* 4.1.4/4.1.3
   Source: Huffman (1994), pages 732–739.

9. **B** *Level:* Application *Competency:* 4.1.4/4.1.3
   Source: Huffman (1994), pages 732–739.

10. **A** *Level:* Application *Competency:* 3.1.10
    Source: Huffman (1994), pages 732–739.

11. **A** *Level:* Application *Competency:* 3.1.10
    Source: Huffman (1994), pages 732–739.

12. **C** *Level:* Application *Competency:* 3.1.10
    Source: Huffman (1994), pages 732–739.

13. **C** *Level:* Application *Competency:* 4.1.4/4.1.3
    Source: Huffman (1994), pages 739–743.

14. **C** *Level:* Application   *Competency:* 4.1.4/4.1.3
    Source: Huffman (1994), pages 739–743.

15. **B** *Level:* Application   *Competency:* 3.1.4
    Source: Huffman (1994), pages 723–725.

16. **B** *Level:* Application   *Competency:* 3.1.4
    Source: Huffman (1994), pages 723–725.

17. **D** *Level:* Knowledge   *Competency:* 4.1.4/4.1.3
    Source: Huffman (1994), pages 739–743.

18. **C** *Level:* Application   *Competency:* 3.1.3
    Source: Rakich et al.(1992), pages 672–674.

19. **C** *Level:* Knowledge   *Competency:* 3.1.10
    Source: Huffman (1994), pages 736–739.

20. **B** *Level:* Application   *Competency:* 3.1.10
    Source: Huffman (1994), pages 736–739.

Human Resource Management References for Further Study

Huffman, E. K. (1994). *Health information management* (10th ed.). Berwyn, IL: Physicians' Record Company.

Kallaus, N. F. & Keeling, B. L. (1991). *Administrative office management* (10th ed.). Cincinnati, OH: South-Western Publishing Co.

Longest, B. (1990). *Management practices for the health professional.* Norwalk, CT: Appleton & Lange.

Rakich, J. S., Longest, B. B., & Darr, K. (1992). *Managing health services organizations* (3rd ed.). Baltimore, MD: Health Professions Press.

Appendices

Appendix I

Medical Record Administrator Entry-Level Domains, Tasks, and Competencies

Domain 1: Assess institutional and patient-related information needs and department (i.e., medical record, quality assurance, cancer registry, or similar department) informational, service, and operational needs.

Task 1.1: Gather data to support patient-related information system needs and departmental operations and services.

Competencies

    1.1.1 Conduct surveys of patients, users of data, health-care providers, administrators, and researchers.
    1.1.2 Conduct interviews with users of data, health-care providers, administrators, researchers, and others.
    1.1.3 Tabulate requests for patient-related data.
    1.1.4 Monitor changes in federal, state, and local laws, regulations, or Joint Commission standards.
    1.1.5 Monitor departmental productivity.
    1.1.6 Collect data on employee performance.
    1.1.7 Compare claims submitted to third-party payers with reimbursement received.
    1.1.8 Monitor work flow under your span of control.

Appendix I

1.1.9   Collect data on the quality of documentation in the medical record (i.e., timeliness, completeness, accuracy).
1.1.10 Tabulate data on the appropriateness and quality of patient care as documented in the medical record (i.e., quality assurance, utilization review activities).
1.1.11 Collect data on the status of incomplete records.
1.1.12 Track location of medical records.
1.1.13 Monitor employee staffing levels.
1.1.14 Monitor accreditation/licensing survey results (i.e., Joint Commission, Medicare, etc.).
1.1.15 Monitor the release of information to ensure confidentiality of patient-related data.
1.1.16 Abstract information from patient records (concurrently or retrospectively) for quality assurance studies, utilization review, or risk management.
1.1.17 Release patient-related data (i.e., reimbursement, research, legal, or patient-related purposes).
1.1.18 Design forms for collection of patient-related or other data (i.e., medical record forms, quality assurance, utilization review forms, etc.).
1.1.19 Abstract information from patient records (concurrently or retrospectively) for research studies.
1.1.20 Abstract information from patient records (concurrently or retrospectively) for reimbursement.
1.1.21 Abstract information from patient records (concurrently or retrospectively) for disease, procedure, physician, or other indices.
1.1.22 Abstract information from patient records (concurrently or retrospectively) for compilation of registries.
1.1.23 Abstract information from patient records (concurrently or retrospectively) for compilation of vital statistics.
1.1.24 Abstract information from patient records (concurrently or retrospectively) to develop user (i.e., physician) profiles.
1.1.25 Confer with peers, providers, or users of departmental or institutional services.
1.1.26 Perform concurrent medical record review.
1.1.27 Participate in departmental or institutional committees.
1.1.28 Assign severity-of-illness categories.
1.1.29 Assign diagnostic/procedure codes using ICD-9-CM, CPT, HCPCS, DSM, or other coding systems.

Task 1.2: Validate data for patient-related information system needs, or for departmental operations or services.

Competencies

    1.2.1 Verify that data have been obtained from valid sources.
    1.2.2 Verify timeliness, completeness, accuracy, and appropriateness of data sources (patient care, management, billing reports, or databases).
    1.2.3 Compare data with standards (i.e., length-of-stay norms, Medicare mortality rates, departmental productivity standards, etc.).
    1.2.4 Check data for internal consistency.
    1.2.5 Perform edit checks to monitor data accuracy.
    1.2.6 Compare data with other data sources or references to determine consistency.
    1.2.7 Validate diagnostic and procedure coding (i.e., ICD-9-CM, CPT, HCPCS, or other coding systems).
    1.2.8 Validate DRG assignment.

Task 1.3: Analyze data for patient-related information system needs or for departmental operations or services.

Competencies

    1.3.1 Prepare data for analysis (i.e., compile data, develop graphs, tables, etc.).
    1.3.2 Perform departmental/institutional case-mix analysis.
    1.3.3 Analyze patient-care data in relation to institutional performance standards.
    1.3.4 Analyze patient-care/institutional data in relation to regulatory and accreditation standards.
    1.3.5 Analyze employee performance data in relation to departmental/institutional performance standards.
    1.3.6 Analyze physician performance data/profiles in relation to medical staff, institutional, or regulatory or accreditation standards.

1.3.7 Analyze clinical or institutional data in relation to previous or current internal and external patterns to identify trends and patterns.
1.3.8 Calculate institutional statistics (i.e., occupancy rates, census, length of stay).
1.3.9 Apply statistical techniques for analyzing departmental/institutional/patient-related data (i.e., mean, standard deviation, variance, etc.).
1.3.10 Apply statistical techniques for determining data validity and reliability (Chronbach's alpha, etc.).
1.3.11 Analyze case-mix payment rates (i.e., DRG and others) to determine reimbursement optimization.
1.3.12 Analyze results of quality assurance, utilization review, risk management, or research studies.

Domain 2: Design and select departmental service, operational, and information systems for patient-related data.

Task 2.1: Design departmental service and operational systems.

Competencies

2.1.1 Develop departmental plans, goals, and objectives for areas under your span of control.
2.1.2 Determine feasibility and constraints applicable to design/redesign of departmental operational systems (i.e., costs, staffing, space, etc.).
2.1.3 Develop or revise departmental policies.
2.1.4 Develop or revise departmental procedures.
2.1.5 Develop or revise job descriptions.
2.1.6 Establish priorities for design or redesign of operational or information systems.
2.1.7 Pilot test new or revised systems.
2.1.8 Develop transition plans for implementation of new or revised systems.
2.1.9 Prepare budgets.
2.1.10 Design departmental operational systems for collection and processing of patient-related data (i.e., quantitative analysis, diagnostic and procedure coding, registries, etc.).

2.1.11 Design departmental operational systems for production control (i.e., establishing productivity levels, production monitoring, etc.).
2.1.12 Design departmental operational systems for information control (i.e., release of patient-related data, record tracking, etc.).
2.1.13 Design departmental operational systems for quality control (i.e., quality control of filing, coding, transcription, etc.).
2.1.14 Design departmental operational systems for information retention and retrieval (i.e., filing systems, filing equipment, retention policies/procedures, etc.).
2.1.15 Design ergonomically sound work environment.
2.1.16 Develop goals and objectives for computerized information systems (i.e., department or other facility systems).
2.1.17 Write functional specification for computerized information systems (i.e., departmental or other facility systems).
2.1.18 Plan computerized system testing procedures (audit scripts) for computerized information systems (departmental or other systems).
2.1.19 Develop computerized system security procedures for computerized information systems (i.e., departmental or other systems).
2.1.20 Develop in-service education programs for departmental or non-departmental staff.

Task 2.2: Identify/select resources to support departmental operations and information systems.

Competencies

2.2.1 Participate in preparation of requests for proposal bids for vendor services.
2.2.2 Evaluate vendor bids.
2.2.3 Review vendor contracts.
2.2.4 Negotiate contracts with vendors.
2.2.5 Prepare requests for proposal for vendor services.
2.2.6 Determine personnel needs for staffing current or new systems.
2.2.7 Determine equipment or supply needs for current or new systems.
2.2.8 Determine space requirements for current or new systems.

Domain 3: Implement departmental service and operational systems, and information systems for patient-related data.

Task 3.1: Execute plan(s) for implementing departmental service and operational systems, and information systems for patient-related data.

Competencies

3.1.1 Select personnel.
3.1.2 Train personnel.
3.1.3 Inform organization staff of plan(s).
3.1.4 Implement new or revised policies and procedures.
3.1.5 Monitor adherence to system specification.
3.1.6 Implement new or revised information, service, or operational systems.
3.1.7 Monitor adherence to budget (i.e., determine budget variance, etc.).
3.1.8 Coordinate on-site review activities (i.e., PRO reviews, etc.).
3.1.9 Monitor policy or procedure compliance.
3.1.10 Counsel or discipline employees.
3.1.11 Terminate employees.
3.1.12 Design employee staffing schedules.
3.1.13 Maintain equipment (i.e., schedule preventive maintenance, arrange for repairs, etc.).
3.1.14 Educate medical record or other students assigned to the facility.
3.1.15 Conduct educational programs for departmental or nondepartmental staff.

Domain 4: Evaluate departmental, operational, and service systems, and information systems for patient-related data.

Task 4.1: Evaluate the effectiveness and efficiency of departmental, operational, and service systems, and information systems for patient-related data.

Competencies

    4.1.1   Monitor system outcomes (i.e., benefits, costs, etc.).
    4.1.2   Determine variation(s) from established objective or standards of performance.
    4.1.3   Recommend changes or improvement(s) in systems.
    4.1.4   Evaluate employee performance.

Appendix II

Medical Record Technician Entry-Level Domains, Tasks, and Competencies

Domain 1: Assess institutional and patient-related information needs and department (i.e., medical record, quality assurance, cancer registry, or similar department) informational, service, and operational needs.

Task 1.1: Gather data to support patient-related information system needs and departmental operations and services.

Competencies

1.1.1 Conduct surveys of patients, users of data, health-care providers, administrators, and researchers.
1.1.2 Conduct interviews with users of data, health-care providers, administrators, researchers, and others.
1.1.3 Tabulate requests for patient-related data.
1.1.4 Monitor changes in federal, state, and local laws, regulations, or Joint Commission standards.
1.1.5 Monitor departmental productivity.
1.1.6 Collect data on employee performance.
1.1.7 Compare claims submitted to third-party payers with reimbursement received.
1.1.8 Monitor work flow under your span of control.

1.1.9 Collect data on the quality of documentation in the medical record (i.e., timeliness, completeness, accuracy).
1.1.10 Tabulate data on the appropriateness and quality of patient care as documented in the medical record (i.e., quality assurance, utilization review activities).
1.1.11 Collect data on the status of incomplete records.
1.1.12 Track location of medical records.
1.1.13 Monitor employee staffing levels.
1.1.14 Monitor accreditation/licensing survey results (i.e., Joint Commission, Medicare, etc.).
1.1.15 Monitor the release of information to ensure confidentiality of patient-related data.
1.1.16 Abstract information from patient records (concurrently or retrospectively) for quality assurance studies, utilization review, or risk management.
1.1.17 Assemble medical records.
1.1.18 Release patient-related data (i.e., reimbursement, research, legal, or patient-related purposes).
1.1.19 Design forms for collection of patient-related or other data (i.e., medical record forms, quality assurance, utilization review forms, etc.).
1.1.20 Abstract information from patient records (concurrently or retrospectively) for research studies.
1.1.21 Abstract information from patient records (concurrently or retrospectively) for reimbursement.
1.1.22 Abstract information from patient records (concurrently or retrospectively) for disease, procedure, physician, or other indices.
1.1.23 Abstract information from patient records (concurrently or retrospectively) for compilation of registries.
1.1.24 Abstract information from patient records (concurrently or retrospectively) for compilation of vital statistics.
1.1.25 Abstract information from patient records (concurrently or retrospectively) to develop user (i.e., physician) profiles.
1.1.26 Confer with peers, providers, or users of departmental or institutional services.
1.1.27 Retrieve or file records.
1.1.28 Perform concurrent medical record review.
1.1.29 Participate in departmental or institutional committees.
1.1.30 Assign severity-of-illness categories.

1.1.31 Assign diagnostic/procedure codes using ICD-9-CM, CPT, HCPCS, DSM, or other coding systems.

Task 1.2: Validate data for patient-related information system needs, or for departmental operations or services.

Competencies

1.2.1 Verify that data have been obtained from valid sources.
1.2.2 Verify timeliness, completeness, accuracy, and appropriateness of data sources (patient care, management, billing reports, or databases).
1.2.3 Compare data with standards (i.e., length-of-stay norms, Medicare mortality rates, departmental productivity standards, etc.).
1.2.4 Check data for internal consistency.
1.2.5 Perform edit checks to monitor data accuracy.
1.2.6 Compare data with other data sources or references to determine consistency.
1.2.7 Validate diagnostic and procedure coding (i.e., ICD-9-CM, CPT, HCPCS, or other coding systems).
1.2.8 Validate DRG assignment.
1.2.9 Validate output on UB-82 or other billing forms.

Task 1.3: Analyze data for patient-related information system needs or for departmental operations or services.

Competencies

1.3.1 Prepare data for analysis (i.e., compile data, develop graphs, tables, etc.).
1.3.2 Perform departmental/institutional case-mix analysis.
1.3.3 Analyze patient care/institutional data in relation to regulatory and accreditation standards.
1.3.4 Analyze employee performance data in relation to departmental/institutional performance standards.

1.3.5 Calculate institutional statistics (i.e., occupancy rates, census, length of stay).
1.3.6 Analyze case-mix payment rates (i.e., DRG and others) to determine reimbursement optimization.

Domain 2: Design and select departmental service, operational, and information systems for patient-related data.

Task 2.1: Design departmental service and operational systems.

Competencies

2.1.1 Develop departmental plans, goals, and objectives for areas under your span of control.
2.1.2 Develop or revise departmental policies.
2.1.3 Develop or revise departmental procedures.
2.1.4 Develop or revise job descriptions.
2.1.5 Develop transition plans for implementation of new or revised systems.
2.1.6 Develop goals and objectives for computerized information systems (i.e., department or other facility systems).
2.1.7 Develop in-service education programs for departmental or non-departmental staff.

Task 2.2: Identify/select resources to support departmental operations and information systems.

Competencies

2.2.1 Determine personnel needs for staffing current or new systems.
2.2.2 Determine equipment or supply needs for current or new systems.
2.2.3 Determine space requirements for current or new systems.

Domain 3: Implement departmental service and operational systems, and information systems for patient-related data.

Task 3.1: Execute plan(s) for implementing departmental service and operational systems, and information systems for patient-related data.

Competencies

- 3.1.1 Select personnel.
- 3.1.2 Train personnel.
- 3.1.3 Inform organization staff of plan(s).
- 3.1.4 Implement new or revised policies and procedures.
- 3.1.5 Monitor adherence to system specification.
- 3.1.6 Implement new or revised information, service, or operational systems.
- 3.1.7 Monitor adherence to budget (i.e., determine budget variance, etc.).
- 3.1.8 Coordinate on-site review activities (i.e., PRO reviews, etc.).
- 3.1.9 Monitor policy or procedure compliance.
- 3.1.10 Counsel or discipline employees.
- 3.1.11 Terminate employees.
- 3.1.12 Design employee staffing schedules.
- 3.1.13 Maintain equipment (i.e., schedule preventive maintenance, arrange for repairs, etc.).
- 3.1.14 Educate medical record or other students assigned to the facility.
- 3.1.15 Conduct educational programs for departmental or nondepartmental staff.

Domain 4: Evaluate departmental, operational, and service systems, and information systems for patient-related data.

Task 4.1: Evaluate the effectiveness and efficiency of departmental, operational, and service systems, and information systems for patient-related data.

Competencies

- 4.1.1 Determine variation(s) from established objective or standards of performance.
- 4.1.2 Recommend changes or improvement(s) in systems.
- 4.1.3 Evaluate employee performance.

Appendix III

MRA and MRT Scoring Grids

MRA Scoring Grid

		Number of Questions					
		Practice Exam 1			**Practice Exam 2**		
		Total	*Correct*	*Score**	*Total*	*Correct*	*Score**
Chapter 2:	The Health Record	20					
Chapter 3:	Retention and Retrieval	20					
Chapter 4:	Health Information Systems	17					
Chapter 5:	Health-Care Statistics	20					
Chapter 6:	Quality of Health Care	20					
Chapter 7:	Classification Systems	20					
Chapter 8:	Coding	30					
Chapter 9:	Legal Issues	20					
Chapter 10:	Management	25					
Chapter 11:	Human Resource Management	20					
	TOTAL	212					

*Divide the number correct by the total number of questions to determine your score for this chapter.

MRT Scoring Grid

		Number of Questions					
		Practice Exam 1			Practice Exam 2		
		Total	Correct	Score*	Total	Correct	Score*
Chapter 2:	The Health Record	20					
Chapter 3:	Retention and Retrieval	20					
Chapter 4:	Health Information Systems	14					
Chapter 5:	Health-Care Statistics	20					
Chapter 6:	Quality of Health Care	20					
Chapter 7:	Classification Systems	20					
Chapter 8:	Coding	30					
Chapter 9:	Legal Issues	20					
Chapter 10:	Management	25					
Chapter 11:	Human Resource Management	20					
	TOTAL	209					

*Divide the number correct by the total number of questions to determine your score for this chapter.

Answer Sheets

Two complete sets of answer sheets for the MRA and MRT practice exams follow. Use the sheets for Practice Exam I the first time you take the exam included in this book. If you are taking the MRA practice exam, the answer sheets are printed on the odd-numbered pages. If you are taking the MRT practice exam, the answer sheets are printed on the even-numbered pages. All answer sheets are clearly marked with the examination title, chapter number, and chapter title. Use the answer sheets for Practice Exam II the second time you take the exam included in this book. Remember to keep track of your scores using the Scoring Grid included in Appendix III.

Practice Exam I Answer Sheets for the MRA and MRT Examinations

Practice Exam I

Date _____

MRA Answer Sheet
Chapter 2
The Health Record

INSTRUCTIONS: Use a #2 pencil and completely darken the circle containing your answer choice for each question. Erase completely to change.

1. C
2. D – C
3. B
4. A
5. B
6. A – D
7. C
8. A
9. C
10. A
11. B
12. B – A
13. A
14. A – C
15. A – B
16. C
17. B – D
18. D
19. D
20. B – C

Practice Exam I

Date _____

MRT Answer Sheet
Chapter 2
The Health Record

INSTRUCTIONS: Use a #2 pencil and completely darken the circle containing your answer choice for each question. Erase completely to change.

1. Ⓐ Ⓑ Ⓒ Ⓓ
2. Ⓐ Ⓑ Ⓒ Ⓓ
3. Ⓐ Ⓑ Ⓒ Ⓓ
4. Ⓐ Ⓑ Ⓒ Ⓓ
5. Ⓐ Ⓑ Ⓒ Ⓓ
6. Ⓐ Ⓑ Ⓒ Ⓓ
7. Ⓐ Ⓑ Ⓒ Ⓓ
8. Ⓐ Ⓑ Ⓒ Ⓓ
9. Ⓐ Ⓑ Ⓒ Ⓓ
10. Ⓐ Ⓑ Ⓒ Ⓓ
11. Ⓐ Ⓑ Ⓒ Ⓓ
12. Ⓐ Ⓑ Ⓒ Ⓓ
13. Ⓐ Ⓑ Ⓒ Ⓓ
14. Ⓐ Ⓑ Ⓒ Ⓓ
15. Ⓐ Ⓑ Ⓒ Ⓓ
16. Ⓐ Ⓑ Ⓒ Ⓓ
17. Ⓐ Ⓑ Ⓒ Ⓓ
18. Ⓐ Ⓑ Ⓒ Ⓓ
19. Ⓐ Ⓑ Ⓒ Ⓓ
20. Ⓐ Ⓑ Ⓒ Ⓓ

Practice Exam I

Date _____

MRA Answer Sheet
Chapter 3
Retention and Retrieval

INSTRUCTIONS: Use a #2 pencil and completely darken the circle containing your answer choice for each question. Erase completely to change.

1. Ⓐ Ⓑ Ⓒ Ⓓ
2. Ⓐ Ⓑ Ⓒ Ⓓ
3. Ⓐ Ⓑ Ⓒ Ⓓ
4. Ⓐ Ⓑ Ⓒ Ⓓ
5. Ⓐ Ⓑ Ⓒ Ⓓ
6. Ⓐ Ⓑ Ⓒ Ⓓ
7. Ⓐ Ⓑ Ⓒ Ⓓ
8. Ⓐ Ⓑ Ⓒ Ⓓ
9. Ⓐ Ⓑ Ⓒ Ⓓ
10. Ⓐ Ⓑ Ⓒ Ⓓ
11. Ⓐ Ⓑ Ⓒ Ⓓ
12. Ⓐ Ⓑ Ⓒ Ⓓ
13. Ⓐ Ⓑ Ⓒ Ⓓ
14. Ⓐ Ⓑ Ⓒ Ⓓ
15. Ⓐ Ⓑ Ⓒ Ⓓ
16. Ⓐ Ⓑ Ⓒ Ⓓ
17. Ⓐ Ⓑ Ⓒ Ⓓ
18. Ⓐ Ⓑ Ⓒ Ⓓ
19. Ⓐ Ⓑ Ⓒ Ⓓ
20. Ⓐ Ⓑ Ⓒ Ⓓ

Practice Exam I

Date _____

MRT Answer Sheet
Chapter 3
Retention and Retrieval

INSTRUCTIONS: Use a #2 pencil and completely darken the circle containing your answer choice for each question. Erase completely to change.

1. Ⓐ Ⓑ Ⓒ Ⓓ
2. Ⓐ Ⓑ Ⓒ Ⓓ
3. Ⓐ Ⓑ Ⓒ Ⓓ
4. Ⓐ Ⓑ Ⓒ Ⓓ
5. Ⓐ Ⓑ Ⓒ Ⓓ
6. Ⓐ Ⓑ Ⓒ Ⓓ
7. Ⓐ Ⓑ Ⓒ Ⓓ
8. Ⓐ Ⓑ Ⓒ Ⓓ
9. Ⓐ Ⓑ Ⓒ Ⓓ
10. Ⓐ Ⓑ Ⓒ Ⓓ
11. Ⓐ Ⓑ Ⓒ Ⓓ
12. Ⓐ Ⓑ Ⓒ Ⓓ
13. Ⓐ Ⓑ Ⓒ Ⓓ
14. Ⓐ Ⓑ Ⓒ Ⓓ
15. Ⓐ Ⓑ Ⓒ Ⓓ
16. Ⓐ Ⓑ Ⓒ Ⓓ
17. Ⓐ Ⓑ Ⓒ Ⓓ
18. Ⓐ Ⓑ Ⓒ Ⓓ
19. Ⓐ Ⓑ Ⓒ Ⓓ
20. Ⓐ Ⓑ Ⓒ Ⓓ

Practice Exam I

Date _____

MRA Answer Sheet
Chapter 4
Health Information Systems

INSTRUCTIONS: Use a #2 pencil and completely darken the circle containing your answer choice for each question. Erase completely to change.

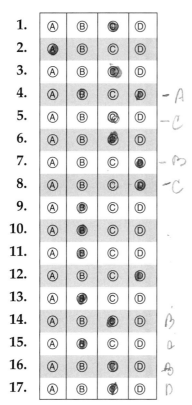

1. C
2. A
3. C
4. D — A
5. C — C
6. C
7. D — B
8. D — C
9. B
10. B
11. B
12. D
13. B
14. C   B
15. B   a
16. C   A
17. C   D

Practice Exam I

Date _____

MRT Answer Sheet
Chapter 4
Health Information Systems

INSTRUCTIONS: Use a #2 pencil and completely darken the circle containing your answer choice for each question. Erase completely to change.

#	A	B	C	D
1.	Ⓐ	Ⓑ	Ⓒ	Ⓓ
2.	Ⓐ	Ⓑ	Ⓒ	Ⓓ
3.	Ⓐ	Ⓑ	Ⓒ	Ⓓ
4.	Ⓐ	Ⓑ	Ⓒ	Ⓓ
5.	Ⓐ	Ⓑ	Ⓒ	Ⓓ
6.	Ⓐ	Ⓑ	Ⓒ	Ⓓ
7.	Ⓐ	Ⓑ	Ⓒ	Ⓓ
8.	Ⓐ	Ⓑ	Ⓒ	Ⓓ
9.	Ⓐ	Ⓑ	Ⓒ	Ⓓ
10.	Ⓐ	Ⓑ	Ⓒ	Ⓓ
11.	Ⓐ	Ⓑ	Ⓒ	Ⓓ
12.	Ⓐ	Ⓑ	Ⓒ	Ⓓ
13.	Ⓐ	Ⓑ	Ⓒ	Ⓓ
14.	Ⓐ	Ⓑ	Ⓒ	Ⓓ

Practice Exam I

Date _____

MRA Answer Sheet
Chapter 5
Health-Care Statistics

INSTRUCTIONS: Use a #2 pencil and completely darken the circle containing your answer choice for each question. Erase completely to change.

1. Ⓐ Ⓑ Ⓒ Ⓓ
2. Ⓐ Ⓑ Ⓒ Ⓓ
3. Ⓐ Ⓑ Ⓒ Ⓓ
4. Ⓐ Ⓑ Ⓒ Ⓓ
5. Ⓐ Ⓑ Ⓒ Ⓓ
6. Ⓐ Ⓑ Ⓒ Ⓓ
7. Ⓐ Ⓑ Ⓒ Ⓓ
8. Ⓐ Ⓑ Ⓒ Ⓓ
9. Ⓐ Ⓑ Ⓒ Ⓓ
10. Ⓐ Ⓑ Ⓒ Ⓓ
11. Ⓐ Ⓑ Ⓒ Ⓓ
12. Ⓐ Ⓑ Ⓒ Ⓓ
13. Ⓐ Ⓑ Ⓒ Ⓓ
14. Ⓐ Ⓑ Ⓒ Ⓓ
15. Ⓐ Ⓑ Ⓒ Ⓓ
16. Ⓐ Ⓑ Ⓒ Ⓓ
17. Ⓐ Ⓑ Ⓒ Ⓓ
18. Ⓐ Ⓑ Ⓒ Ⓓ
19. Ⓐ Ⓑ Ⓒ Ⓓ
20. Ⓐ Ⓑ Ⓒ Ⓓ

Practice Exam I

Date _____

MRT Answer Sheet
Chapter 5
Health-Care Statistics

INSTRUCTIONS: Use a #2 pencil and completely darken the circle containing your answer choice for each question. Erase completely to change.

1. Ⓐ Ⓑ Ⓒ Ⓓ
2. Ⓐ Ⓑ Ⓒ Ⓓ
3. Ⓐ Ⓑ Ⓒ Ⓓ
4. Ⓐ Ⓑ Ⓒ Ⓓ
5. Ⓐ Ⓑ Ⓒ Ⓓ
6. Ⓐ Ⓑ Ⓒ Ⓓ
7. Ⓐ Ⓑ Ⓒ Ⓓ
8. Ⓐ Ⓑ Ⓒ Ⓓ
9. Ⓐ Ⓑ Ⓒ Ⓓ
10. Ⓐ Ⓑ Ⓒ Ⓓ
11. Ⓐ Ⓑ Ⓒ Ⓓ
12. Ⓐ Ⓑ Ⓒ Ⓓ
13. Ⓐ Ⓑ Ⓒ Ⓓ
14. Ⓐ Ⓑ Ⓒ Ⓓ
15. Ⓐ Ⓑ Ⓒ Ⓓ
16. Ⓐ Ⓑ Ⓒ Ⓓ
17. Ⓐ Ⓑ Ⓒ Ⓓ
18. Ⓐ Ⓑ Ⓒ Ⓓ
19. Ⓐ Ⓑ Ⓒ Ⓓ
20. Ⓐ Ⓑ Ⓒ Ⓓ

Practice Exam I

Date _____

MRA Answer Sheet
Chapter 6
Quality of Health Care

INSTRUCTIONS: Use a #2 pencil and completely darken the circle containing your answer choice for each question. Erase completely to change.

1. Ⓐ Ⓑ Ⓒ Ⓓ
2. Ⓐ Ⓑ Ⓒ Ⓓ
3. Ⓐ Ⓑ Ⓒ Ⓓ
4. Ⓐ Ⓑ Ⓒ Ⓓ
5. Ⓐ Ⓑ Ⓒ Ⓓ
6. Ⓐ Ⓑ Ⓒ Ⓓ
7. Ⓐ Ⓑ Ⓒ Ⓓ
8. Ⓐ Ⓑ Ⓒ Ⓓ
9. Ⓐ Ⓑ Ⓒ Ⓓ
10. Ⓐ Ⓑ Ⓒ Ⓓ
11. Ⓐ Ⓑ Ⓒ Ⓓ
12. Ⓐ Ⓑ Ⓒ Ⓓ
13. Ⓐ Ⓑ Ⓒ Ⓓ
14. Ⓐ Ⓑ Ⓒ Ⓓ
15. Ⓐ Ⓑ Ⓒ Ⓓ
16. Ⓐ Ⓑ Ⓒ Ⓓ
17. Ⓐ Ⓑ Ⓒ Ⓓ
18. Ⓐ Ⓑ Ⓒ Ⓓ
19. Ⓐ Ⓑ Ⓒ Ⓓ
20. Ⓐ Ⓑ Ⓒ Ⓓ

Practice Exam I

Date _____

MRT Answer Sheet
Chapter 6
Quality of Health Care

INSTRUCTIONS: Use a #2 pencil and completely darken the circle containing your answer choice for each question. Erase completely to change.

1. Ⓐ Ⓑ Ⓒ Ⓓ
2. Ⓐ Ⓑ Ⓒ Ⓓ
3. Ⓐ Ⓑ Ⓒ Ⓓ
4. Ⓐ Ⓑ Ⓒ Ⓓ
5. Ⓐ Ⓑ Ⓒ Ⓓ
6. Ⓐ Ⓑ Ⓒ Ⓓ
7. Ⓐ Ⓑ Ⓒ Ⓓ
8. Ⓐ Ⓑ Ⓒ Ⓓ
9. Ⓐ Ⓑ Ⓒ Ⓓ
10. Ⓐ Ⓑ Ⓒ Ⓓ
11. Ⓐ Ⓑ Ⓒ Ⓓ
12. Ⓐ Ⓑ Ⓒ Ⓓ
13. Ⓐ Ⓑ Ⓒ Ⓓ
14. Ⓐ Ⓑ Ⓒ Ⓓ
15. Ⓐ Ⓑ Ⓒ Ⓓ
16. Ⓐ Ⓑ Ⓒ Ⓓ
17. Ⓐ Ⓑ Ⓒ Ⓓ
18. Ⓐ Ⓑ Ⓒ Ⓓ
19. Ⓐ Ⓑ Ⓒ Ⓓ
20. Ⓐ Ⓑ Ⓒ Ⓓ

Practice Exam I

Date _____

MRA Answer Sheet
Chapter 7
Classification Systems

INSTRUCTIONS: Use a #2 pencil and completely darken the circle containing your answer choice for each question. Erase completely to change.

1. Ⓐ Ⓑ Ⓒ Ⓓ
2. **Ⓐ** Ⓑ Ⓒ Ⓓ
3. Ⓐ Ⓑ Ⓒ Ⓓ
4. **Ⓐ** Ⓑ Ⓒ Ⓓ
5. Ⓐ Ⓑ Ⓒ Ⓓ
6. **Ⓐ** Ⓑ Ⓒ Ⓓ
7. Ⓐ Ⓑ Ⓒ Ⓓ
8. **Ⓐ** Ⓑ Ⓒ Ⓓ
9. Ⓐ Ⓑ Ⓒ Ⓓ
10. **Ⓐ** Ⓑ Ⓒ Ⓓ
11. Ⓐ Ⓑ Ⓒ Ⓓ
12. **Ⓐ** Ⓑ Ⓒ Ⓓ
13. Ⓐ Ⓑ Ⓒ Ⓓ
14. **Ⓐ** Ⓑ Ⓒ Ⓓ
15. Ⓐ Ⓑ Ⓒ Ⓓ
16. **Ⓐ** Ⓑ Ⓒ Ⓓ
17. Ⓐ Ⓑ Ⓒ Ⓓ
18. **Ⓐ** Ⓑ Ⓒ Ⓓ
19. Ⓐ Ⓑ Ⓒ Ⓓ
20. **Ⓐ** Ⓑ Ⓒ Ⓓ

Practice Exam I

Date _____

MRT Answer Sheet
Chapter 7
Classification Systems

INSTRUCTIONS: Use a #2 pencil and completely darken the circle containing your answer choice for each question. Erase completely to change.

1. Ⓐ Ⓑ Ⓒ Ⓓ
2. Ⓐ Ⓑ Ⓒ Ⓓ
3. Ⓐ Ⓑ Ⓒ Ⓓ
4. Ⓐ Ⓑ Ⓒ Ⓓ
5. Ⓐ Ⓑ Ⓒ Ⓓ
6. Ⓐ Ⓑ Ⓒ Ⓓ
7. Ⓐ Ⓑ Ⓒ Ⓓ
8. Ⓐ Ⓑ Ⓒ Ⓓ
9. Ⓐ Ⓑ Ⓒ Ⓓ
10. Ⓐ Ⓑ Ⓒ Ⓓ
11. Ⓐ Ⓑ Ⓒ Ⓓ
12. Ⓐ Ⓑ Ⓒ Ⓓ
13. Ⓐ Ⓑ Ⓒ Ⓓ

Practice Exam I

Date _____

MRA Answer Sheet
Chapter 8
Coding

INSTRUCTIONS: Use a #2 pencil and completely darken the circle containing your answer choice for each question. Erase completely to change.

#	A	B	C	D		#	A	B	C	D
1.	Ⓐ	Ⓑ	Ⓒ	Ⓓ		16.	Ⓐ	Ⓑ	Ⓒ	Ⓓ
2.	Ⓐ	Ⓑ	Ⓒ	Ⓓ		17.	Ⓐ	Ⓑ	Ⓒ	Ⓓ
3.	Ⓐ	Ⓑ	Ⓒ	Ⓓ		18.	Ⓐ	Ⓑ	Ⓒ	Ⓓ
4.	Ⓐ	Ⓑ	Ⓒ	Ⓓ		19.	Ⓐ	Ⓑ	Ⓒ	Ⓓ
5.	Ⓐ	Ⓑ	Ⓒ	Ⓓ		20.	Ⓐ	Ⓑ	Ⓒ	Ⓓ
6.	Ⓐ	Ⓑ	Ⓒ	Ⓓ		21.	Ⓐ	Ⓑ	Ⓒ	Ⓓ
7.	Ⓐ	Ⓑ	Ⓒ	Ⓓ		22.	Ⓐ	Ⓑ	Ⓒ	Ⓓ
8.	Ⓐ	Ⓑ	Ⓒ	Ⓓ		23.	Ⓐ	Ⓑ	Ⓒ	Ⓓ
9.	Ⓐ	Ⓑ	Ⓒ	Ⓓ		24.	Ⓐ	Ⓑ	Ⓒ	Ⓓ
10.	Ⓐ	Ⓑ	Ⓒ	Ⓓ		25.	Ⓐ	Ⓑ	Ⓒ	Ⓓ
11.	Ⓐ	Ⓑ	Ⓒ	Ⓓ		26.	Ⓐ	Ⓑ	Ⓒ	Ⓓ
12.	Ⓐ	Ⓑ	Ⓒ	Ⓓ		27.	Ⓐ	Ⓑ	Ⓒ	Ⓓ
13.	Ⓐ	Ⓑ	Ⓒ	Ⓓ		28.	Ⓐ	Ⓑ	Ⓒ	Ⓓ
14.	Ⓐ	Ⓑ	Ⓒ	Ⓓ		29.	Ⓐ	Ⓑ	Ⓒ	Ⓓ
15.	Ⓐ	Ⓑ	Ⓒ	Ⓓ		30.	Ⓐ	Ⓑ	Ⓒ	Ⓓ

Practice Exam I

Date _____

MRT Answer Sheet
Chapter 8
Coding

INSTRUCTIONS: Use a #2 pencil and completely darken the circle containing your answer choice for each question. Erase completely to change.

	A	B	C	D			A	B	C	D
1.	Ⓐ	Ⓑ	Ⓒ	Ⓓ		16.	Ⓐ	Ⓑ	Ⓒ	Ⓓ
2.	Ⓐ	Ⓑ	Ⓒ	Ⓓ		17.	Ⓐ	Ⓑ	Ⓒ	Ⓓ
3.	Ⓐ	Ⓑ	Ⓒ	Ⓓ		18.	Ⓐ	Ⓑ	Ⓒ	Ⓓ
4.	Ⓐ	Ⓑ	Ⓒ	Ⓓ		19.	Ⓐ	Ⓑ	Ⓒ	Ⓓ
5.	Ⓐ	Ⓑ	Ⓒ	Ⓓ		20.	Ⓐ	Ⓑ	Ⓒ	Ⓓ
6.	Ⓐ	Ⓑ	Ⓒ	Ⓓ		21.	Ⓐ	Ⓑ	Ⓒ	Ⓓ
7.	Ⓐ	Ⓑ	Ⓒ	Ⓓ		22.	Ⓐ	Ⓑ	Ⓒ	Ⓓ
8.	Ⓐ	Ⓑ	Ⓒ	Ⓓ		23.	Ⓐ	Ⓑ	Ⓒ	Ⓓ
9.	Ⓐ	Ⓑ	Ⓒ	Ⓓ		24.	Ⓐ	Ⓑ	Ⓒ	Ⓓ
10.	Ⓐ	Ⓑ	Ⓒ	Ⓓ		25.	Ⓐ	Ⓑ	Ⓒ	Ⓓ
11.	Ⓐ	Ⓑ	Ⓒ	Ⓓ		26.	Ⓐ	Ⓑ	Ⓒ	Ⓓ
12.	Ⓐ	Ⓑ	Ⓒ	Ⓓ		27.	Ⓐ	Ⓑ	Ⓒ	Ⓓ
13.	Ⓐ	Ⓑ	Ⓒ	Ⓓ		28.	Ⓐ	Ⓑ	Ⓒ	Ⓓ
14.	Ⓐ	Ⓑ	Ⓒ	Ⓓ		29.	Ⓐ	Ⓑ	Ⓒ	Ⓓ
15.	Ⓐ	Ⓑ	Ⓒ	Ⓓ		30.	Ⓐ	Ⓑ	Ⓒ	Ⓓ

Practice Exam I

Date _____

MRA Answer Sheet
Chapter 9
Legal Issues

INSTRUCTIONS: Use a #2 pencil and completely darken the circle containing your answer choice for each question. Erase completely to change.

1. Ⓐ Ⓑ Ⓒ Ⓓ
2. Ⓐ Ⓑ Ⓒ Ⓓ
3. Ⓐ Ⓑ Ⓒ Ⓓ
4. Ⓐ Ⓑ Ⓒ Ⓓ
5. Ⓐ Ⓑ Ⓒ Ⓓ
6. Ⓐ Ⓑ Ⓒ Ⓓ
7. Ⓐ Ⓑ Ⓒ Ⓓ
8. Ⓐ Ⓑ Ⓒ Ⓓ
9. Ⓐ Ⓑ Ⓒ Ⓓ
10. Ⓐ Ⓑ Ⓒ Ⓓ
11. Ⓐ Ⓑ Ⓒ Ⓓ
12. Ⓐ Ⓑ Ⓒ Ⓓ
13. Ⓐ Ⓑ Ⓒ Ⓓ
14. Ⓐ Ⓑ Ⓒ Ⓓ
15. Ⓐ Ⓑ Ⓒ Ⓓ
16. Ⓐ Ⓑ Ⓒ Ⓓ
17. Ⓐ Ⓑ Ⓒ Ⓓ
18. Ⓐ Ⓑ Ⓒ Ⓓ
19. Ⓐ Ⓑ Ⓒ Ⓓ
20. Ⓐ Ⓑ Ⓒ Ⓓ

Practice Exam I

Date _____

MRT Answer Sheet
Chapter 9
Legal Issues

INSTRUCTIONS: Use a #2 pencil and completely darken the circle containing your answer choice for each question. Erase completely to change.

1. Ⓐ Ⓑ Ⓒ Ⓓ
2. Ⓐ Ⓑ Ⓒ Ⓓ
3. Ⓐ Ⓑ Ⓒ Ⓓ
4. Ⓐ Ⓑ Ⓒ Ⓓ
5. Ⓐ Ⓑ Ⓒ Ⓓ
6. Ⓐ Ⓑ Ⓒ Ⓓ
7. Ⓐ Ⓑ Ⓒ Ⓓ
8. Ⓐ Ⓑ Ⓒ Ⓓ
9. Ⓐ Ⓑ Ⓒ Ⓓ
10. Ⓐ Ⓑ Ⓒ Ⓓ
11. Ⓐ Ⓑ Ⓒ Ⓓ
12. Ⓐ Ⓑ Ⓒ Ⓓ
13. Ⓐ Ⓑ Ⓒ Ⓓ
14. Ⓐ Ⓑ Ⓒ Ⓓ
15. Ⓐ Ⓑ Ⓒ Ⓓ
16. Ⓐ Ⓑ Ⓒ Ⓓ
17. Ⓐ Ⓑ Ⓒ Ⓓ
18. Ⓐ Ⓑ Ⓒ Ⓓ
19. Ⓐ Ⓑ Ⓒ Ⓓ
20. Ⓐ Ⓑ Ⓒ Ⓓ

Practice Exam I

Date _____

MRA Answer Sheet
Chapter 10
Management

INSTRUCTIONS: Use a #2 pencil and completely darken the circle containing your answer choice for each question. Erase completely to change.

	A	B	C	D			A	B	C	D
1.	Ⓐ	Ⓑ	Ⓒ	Ⓓ		16.	Ⓐ	Ⓑ	Ⓒ	Ⓓ
2.	Ⓐ	Ⓑ	Ⓒ	Ⓓ		17.	Ⓐ	Ⓑ	Ⓒ	Ⓓ
3.	Ⓐ	Ⓑ	Ⓒ	Ⓓ		18.	Ⓐ	Ⓑ	Ⓒ	Ⓓ
4.	Ⓐ	Ⓑ	Ⓒ	Ⓓ		19.	Ⓐ	Ⓑ	Ⓒ	Ⓓ
5.	Ⓐ	Ⓑ	Ⓒ	Ⓓ		20.	Ⓐ	Ⓑ	Ⓒ	Ⓓ
6.	Ⓐ	Ⓑ	Ⓒ	Ⓓ		21.	Ⓐ	Ⓑ	Ⓒ	Ⓓ
7.	Ⓐ	Ⓑ	Ⓒ	Ⓓ		22.	Ⓐ	Ⓑ	Ⓒ	Ⓓ
8.	Ⓐ	Ⓑ	Ⓒ	Ⓓ		23.	Ⓐ	Ⓑ	Ⓒ	Ⓓ
9.	Ⓐ	Ⓑ	Ⓒ	Ⓓ		24.	Ⓐ	Ⓑ	Ⓒ	Ⓓ
10.	Ⓐ	Ⓑ	Ⓒ	Ⓓ		25.	Ⓐ	Ⓑ	Ⓒ	Ⓓ
11.	Ⓐ	Ⓑ	Ⓒ	Ⓓ						
12.	Ⓐ	Ⓑ	Ⓒ	Ⓓ						
13.	Ⓐ	Ⓑ	Ⓒ	Ⓓ						
14.	Ⓐ	Ⓑ	Ⓒ	Ⓓ						
15.	Ⓐ	Ⓑ	Ⓒ	Ⓓ						

Practice Exam I

Date _____

MRT Answer Sheet
Chapter 10
Management

INSTRUCTIONS: Use a #2 pencil and completely darken the circle containing your answer choice for each question. Erase completely to change.

#	A	B	C	D		#	A	B	C	D
1.	Ⓐ	Ⓑ	Ⓒ	Ⓓ		16.	Ⓐ	Ⓑ	Ⓒ	Ⓓ
2.	Ⓐ	Ⓑ	Ⓒ	Ⓓ		17.	Ⓐ	Ⓑ	Ⓒ	Ⓓ
3.	Ⓐ	Ⓑ	Ⓒ	Ⓓ		18.	Ⓐ	Ⓑ	Ⓒ	Ⓓ
4.	Ⓐ	Ⓑ	Ⓒ	Ⓓ		19.	Ⓐ	Ⓑ	Ⓒ	Ⓓ
5.	Ⓐ	Ⓑ	Ⓒ	Ⓓ		20.	Ⓐ	Ⓑ	Ⓒ	Ⓓ
6.	Ⓐ	Ⓑ	Ⓒ	Ⓓ		21.	Ⓐ	Ⓑ	Ⓒ	Ⓓ
7.	Ⓐ	Ⓑ	Ⓒ	Ⓓ		22.	Ⓐ	Ⓑ	Ⓒ	Ⓓ
8.	Ⓐ	Ⓑ	Ⓒ	Ⓓ		23.	Ⓐ	Ⓑ	Ⓒ	Ⓓ
9.	Ⓐ	Ⓑ	Ⓒ	Ⓓ		24.	Ⓐ	Ⓑ	Ⓒ	Ⓓ
10.	Ⓐ	Ⓑ	Ⓒ	Ⓓ		25.	Ⓐ	Ⓑ	Ⓒ	Ⓓ
11.	Ⓐ	Ⓑ	Ⓒ	Ⓓ						
12.	Ⓐ	Ⓑ	Ⓒ	Ⓓ						
13.	Ⓐ	Ⓑ	Ⓒ	Ⓓ						
14.	Ⓐ	Ⓑ	Ⓒ	Ⓓ						
15.	Ⓐ	Ⓑ	Ⓒ	Ⓓ						

Practice Exam I

Date _____

MRA Answer Sheet
Chapter 11
Human Resource Management

INSTRUCTIONS: Use a #2 pencil and completely darken the circle containing your answer choice for each question. Erase completely to change.

1. Ⓐ Ⓑ Ⓒ Ⓓ
2. Ⓐ Ⓑ Ⓒ Ⓓ
3. Ⓐ Ⓑ Ⓒ Ⓓ
4. Ⓐ Ⓑ Ⓒ Ⓓ
5. Ⓐ Ⓑ Ⓒ Ⓓ
6. Ⓐ Ⓑ Ⓒ Ⓓ
7. Ⓐ Ⓑ Ⓒ Ⓓ
8. Ⓐ Ⓑ Ⓒ Ⓓ
9. Ⓐ Ⓑ Ⓒ Ⓓ
10. Ⓐ Ⓑ Ⓒ Ⓓ
11. Ⓐ Ⓑ Ⓒ Ⓓ
12. Ⓐ Ⓑ Ⓒ Ⓓ
13. Ⓐ Ⓑ Ⓒ Ⓓ
14. Ⓐ Ⓑ Ⓒ Ⓓ
15. Ⓐ Ⓑ Ⓒ Ⓓ
16. Ⓐ Ⓑ Ⓒ Ⓓ
17. Ⓐ Ⓑ Ⓒ Ⓓ
18. Ⓐ Ⓑ Ⓒ Ⓓ
19. Ⓐ Ⓑ Ⓒ Ⓓ
20. Ⓐ Ⓑ Ⓒ Ⓓ

Practice Exam I

Date _____

MRT Answer Sheet
Chapter 11
Human Resource Management

INSTRUCTIONS: Use a #2 pencil and completely darken the circle containing your answer choice for each question. Erase completely to change.

1. Ⓐ Ⓑ Ⓒ Ⓓ
2. Ⓐ Ⓑ Ⓒ Ⓓ
3. Ⓐ Ⓑ Ⓒ Ⓓ
4. Ⓐ Ⓑ Ⓒ Ⓓ
5. Ⓐ Ⓑ Ⓒ Ⓓ
6. Ⓐ Ⓑ Ⓒ Ⓓ
7. Ⓐ Ⓑ Ⓒ Ⓓ
8. Ⓐ Ⓑ Ⓒ Ⓓ
9. Ⓐ Ⓑ Ⓒ Ⓓ
10. Ⓐ Ⓑ Ⓒ Ⓓ
11. Ⓐ Ⓑ Ⓒ Ⓓ
12. Ⓐ Ⓑ Ⓒ Ⓓ
13. Ⓐ Ⓑ Ⓒ Ⓓ
14. Ⓐ Ⓑ Ⓒ Ⓓ
15. Ⓐ Ⓑ Ⓒ Ⓓ
16. Ⓐ Ⓑ Ⓒ Ⓓ
17. Ⓐ Ⓑ Ⓒ Ⓓ
18. Ⓐ Ⓑ Ⓒ Ⓓ
19. Ⓐ Ⓑ Ⓒ Ⓓ
20. Ⓐ Ⓑ Ⓒ Ⓓ

Practice Exam II Answer Sheets for the MRA and MRT Examinations

Practice Exam II

Date _____

MRA Answer Sheet
Chapter 2
The Health Record

INSTRUCTIONS: Use a #2 pencil and completely darken the circle containing your answer choice for each question. Erase completely to change.

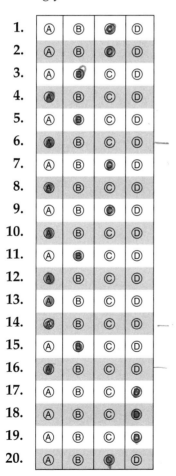

1. C
2. C
3. B
4. A
5. B
6. A
7. C
8. A
9. C
10. A
11. B
12. A
13. A
14. A
15. B
16. A
17. D
18. D
19. D
20. C

Practice Exam II

Date _____

MRT Answer Sheet
Chapter 2
The Health Record

INSTRUCTIONS: Use a #2 pencil and completely darken the circle containing your answer choice for each question. Erase completely to change.

1. Ⓐ Ⓑ Ⓒ Ⓓ
2. Ⓐ Ⓑ Ⓒ Ⓓ
3. Ⓐ Ⓑ Ⓒ Ⓓ
4. Ⓐ Ⓑ Ⓒ Ⓓ
5. Ⓐ Ⓑ Ⓒ Ⓓ
6. Ⓐ Ⓑ Ⓒ Ⓓ
7. Ⓐ Ⓑ Ⓒ Ⓓ
8. Ⓐ Ⓑ Ⓒ Ⓓ
9. Ⓐ Ⓑ Ⓒ Ⓓ
10. Ⓐ Ⓑ Ⓒ Ⓓ
11. Ⓐ Ⓑ Ⓒ Ⓓ
12. Ⓐ Ⓑ Ⓒ Ⓓ
13. Ⓐ Ⓑ Ⓒ Ⓓ
14. Ⓐ Ⓑ Ⓒ Ⓓ
15. Ⓐ Ⓑ Ⓒ Ⓓ
16. Ⓐ Ⓑ Ⓒ Ⓓ
17. Ⓐ Ⓑ Ⓒ Ⓓ
18. Ⓐ Ⓑ Ⓒ Ⓓ
19. Ⓐ Ⓑ Ⓒ Ⓓ
20. Ⓐ Ⓑ Ⓒ Ⓓ

Practice Exam II

Date _____

MRA Answer Sheet
Chapter 3
Retention and Retrieval

INSTRUCTIONS: Use a #2 pencil and completely darken the circle containing your answer choice for each question. Erase completely to change.

1. Ⓐ Ⓑ Ⓒ Ⓓ
2. Ⓐ Ⓑ Ⓒ Ⓓ
3. Ⓐ Ⓑ Ⓒ Ⓓ
4. Ⓐ Ⓑ Ⓒ Ⓓ
5. Ⓐ Ⓑ Ⓒ Ⓓ
6. Ⓐ Ⓑ Ⓒ Ⓓ
7. Ⓐ Ⓑ Ⓒ Ⓓ
8. Ⓐ Ⓑ Ⓒ Ⓓ
9. Ⓐ Ⓑ Ⓒ Ⓓ
10. Ⓐ Ⓑ Ⓒ Ⓓ
11. Ⓐ Ⓑ Ⓒ Ⓓ
12. Ⓐ Ⓑ Ⓒ Ⓓ
13. Ⓐ Ⓑ Ⓒ Ⓓ
14. Ⓐ Ⓑ Ⓒ Ⓓ
15. Ⓐ Ⓑ Ⓒ Ⓓ
16. Ⓐ Ⓑ Ⓒ Ⓓ
17. Ⓐ Ⓑ Ⓒ Ⓓ
18. Ⓐ Ⓑ Ⓒ Ⓓ
19. Ⓐ Ⓑ Ⓒ Ⓓ
20. Ⓐ Ⓑ Ⓒ Ⓓ

Practice Exam II

Date _____

MRT Answer Sheet
Chapter 3
Retention and Retrieval

INSTRUCTIONS: Use a #2 pencil and completely darken the circle containing your answer choice for each question. Erase completely to change.

1. Ⓐ Ⓑ Ⓒ Ⓓ
2. Ⓐ Ⓑ Ⓒ Ⓓ
3. Ⓐ Ⓑ Ⓒ Ⓓ
4. Ⓐ Ⓑ Ⓒ Ⓓ
5. Ⓐ Ⓑ Ⓒ Ⓓ
6. Ⓐ Ⓑ Ⓒ Ⓓ
7. Ⓐ Ⓑ Ⓒ Ⓓ
8. Ⓐ Ⓑ Ⓒ Ⓓ
9. Ⓐ Ⓑ Ⓒ Ⓓ
10. Ⓐ Ⓑ Ⓒ Ⓓ
11. Ⓐ Ⓑ Ⓒ Ⓓ
12. Ⓐ Ⓑ Ⓒ Ⓓ
13. Ⓐ Ⓑ Ⓒ Ⓓ
14. Ⓐ Ⓑ Ⓒ Ⓓ
15. Ⓐ Ⓑ Ⓒ Ⓓ
16. Ⓐ Ⓑ Ⓒ Ⓓ
17. Ⓐ Ⓑ Ⓒ Ⓓ
18. Ⓐ Ⓑ Ⓒ Ⓓ
19. Ⓐ Ⓑ Ⓒ Ⓓ
20. Ⓐ Ⓑ Ⓒ Ⓓ

Practice Exam II

Date _____

MRA Answer Sheet
Chapter 4
Health Information Systems

INSTRUCTIONS: Use a #2 pencil and completely darken the circle containing your answer choice for each question. Erase completely to change.

#	A	B	C	D
1.	Ⓐ	Ⓑ	Ⓒ	Ⓓ
2.	Ⓐ	Ⓑ	Ⓒ	Ⓓ
3.	Ⓐ	Ⓑ	Ⓒ	Ⓓ
4.	Ⓐ	Ⓑ	Ⓒ	Ⓓ
5.	Ⓐ	Ⓑ	Ⓒ	Ⓓ
6.	Ⓐ	Ⓑ	Ⓒ	Ⓓ
7.	Ⓐ	Ⓑ	Ⓒ	Ⓓ
8.	Ⓐ	Ⓑ	Ⓒ	Ⓓ
9.	Ⓐ	Ⓑ	Ⓒ	Ⓓ
10.	Ⓐ	Ⓑ	Ⓒ	Ⓓ
11.	Ⓐ	Ⓑ	Ⓒ	Ⓓ
12.	Ⓐ	Ⓑ	Ⓒ	Ⓓ
13.	Ⓐ	Ⓑ	Ⓒ	Ⓓ
14.	Ⓐ	Ⓑ	Ⓒ	Ⓓ
15.	Ⓐ	Ⓑ	Ⓒ	Ⓓ
16.	Ⓐ	Ⓑ	Ⓒ	Ⓓ
17.	Ⓐ	Ⓑ	Ⓒ	Ⓓ

Practice Exam II

Date _____

MRT Answer Sheet
Chapter 4
Health Information Systems

INSTRUCTIONS: Use a #2 pencil and completely darken the circle containing your answer choice for each question. Erase completely to change.

1. Ⓐ Ⓑ Ⓒ Ⓓ
2. Ⓐ Ⓑ Ⓒ Ⓓ
3. Ⓐ Ⓑ Ⓒ Ⓓ
4. Ⓐ Ⓑ Ⓒ Ⓓ
5. Ⓐ Ⓑ Ⓒ Ⓓ
6. Ⓐ Ⓑ Ⓒ Ⓓ
7. Ⓐ Ⓑ Ⓒ Ⓓ
8. Ⓐ Ⓑ Ⓒ Ⓓ
9. Ⓐ Ⓑ Ⓒ Ⓓ
10. Ⓐ Ⓑ Ⓒ Ⓓ
11. Ⓐ Ⓑ Ⓒ Ⓓ
12. Ⓐ Ⓑ Ⓒ Ⓓ
13. Ⓐ Ⓑ Ⓒ Ⓓ
14. Ⓐ Ⓑ Ⓒ Ⓓ

Practice Exam II

Date _____

MRA Answer Sheet
Chapter 5
Health-Care Statistics

INSTRUCTIONS: Use a #2 pencil and completely darken the circle containing your answer choice for each question. Erase completely to change.

1. Ⓐ Ⓑ Ⓒ Ⓓ
2. Ⓐ Ⓑ Ⓒ Ⓓ
3. Ⓐ Ⓑ Ⓒ Ⓓ
4. Ⓐ Ⓑ Ⓒ Ⓓ
5. Ⓐ Ⓑ Ⓒ Ⓓ
6. Ⓐ Ⓑ Ⓒ Ⓓ
7. Ⓐ Ⓑ Ⓒ Ⓓ
8. Ⓐ Ⓑ Ⓒ Ⓓ
9. Ⓐ Ⓑ Ⓒ Ⓓ
10. Ⓐ Ⓑ Ⓒ Ⓓ
11. Ⓐ Ⓑ Ⓒ Ⓓ
12. Ⓐ Ⓑ Ⓒ Ⓓ
13. Ⓐ Ⓑ Ⓒ Ⓓ
14. Ⓐ Ⓑ Ⓒ Ⓓ
15. Ⓐ Ⓑ Ⓒ Ⓓ
16. Ⓐ Ⓑ Ⓒ Ⓓ
17. Ⓐ Ⓑ Ⓒ Ⓓ
18. Ⓐ Ⓑ Ⓒ Ⓓ
19. Ⓐ Ⓑ Ⓒ Ⓓ
20. Ⓐ Ⓑ Ⓒ Ⓓ

Practice Exam II

Date _____

MRT Answer Sheet
Chapter 5
Health-Care Statistics

INSTRUCTIONS: Use a #2 pencil and completely darken the circle containing your answer choice for each question. Erase completely to change.

1. Ⓐ Ⓑ Ⓒ Ⓓ
2. Ⓐ Ⓑ Ⓒ Ⓓ
3. Ⓐ Ⓑ Ⓒ Ⓓ
4. Ⓐ Ⓑ Ⓒ Ⓓ
5. Ⓐ Ⓑ Ⓒ Ⓓ
6. Ⓐ Ⓑ Ⓒ Ⓓ
7. Ⓐ Ⓑ Ⓒ Ⓓ
8. Ⓐ Ⓑ Ⓒ Ⓓ
9. Ⓐ Ⓑ Ⓒ Ⓓ
10. Ⓐ Ⓑ Ⓒ Ⓓ
11. Ⓐ Ⓑ Ⓒ Ⓓ
12. Ⓐ Ⓑ Ⓒ Ⓓ
13. Ⓐ Ⓑ Ⓒ Ⓓ
14. Ⓐ Ⓑ Ⓒ Ⓓ
15. Ⓐ Ⓑ Ⓒ Ⓓ
16. Ⓐ Ⓑ Ⓒ Ⓓ
17. Ⓐ Ⓑ Ⓒ Ⓓ
18. Ⓐ Ⓑ Ⓒ Ⓓ
19. Ⓐ Ⓑ Ⓒ Ⓓ
20. Ⓐ Ⓑ Ⓒ Ⓓ

Practice Exam II

Date _____

MRA Answer Sheet
Chapter 6
Quality of Health Care

INSTRUCTIONS: Use a #2 pencil and completely darken the circle containing your answer choice for each question. Erase completely to change.

1. Ⓐ Ⓑ Ⓒ Ⓓ
2. Ⓐ Ⓑ Ⓒ Ⓓ
3. Ⓐ Ⓑ Ⓒ Ⓓ
4. Ⓐ Ⓑ Ⓒ Ⓓ
5. Ⓐ Ⓑ Ⓒ Ⓓ
6. Ⓐ Ⓑ Ⓒ Ⓓ
7. Ⓐ Ⓑ Ⓒ Ⓓ
8. Ⓐ Ⓑ Ⓒ Ⓓ
9. Ⓐ Ⓑ Ⓒ Ⓓ
10. Ⓐ Ⓑ Ⓒ Ⓓ
11. Ⓐ Ⓑ Ⓒ Ⓓ
12. Ⓐ Ⓑ Ⓒ Ⓓ
13. Ⓐ Ⓑ Ⓒ Ⓓ
14. Ⓐ Ⓑ Ⓒ Ⓓ
15. Ⓐ Ⓑ Ⓒ Ⓓ
16. Ⓐ Ⓑ Ⓒ Ⓓ
17. Ⓐ Ⓑ Ⓒ Ⓓ
18. Ⓐ Ⓑ Ⓒ Ⓓ
19. Ⓐ Ⓑ Ⓒ Ⓓ
20. Ⓐ Ⓑ Ⓒ Ⓓ

Practice Exam II

Date _____

MRT Answer Sheet
Chapter 6
Quality of Health Care

INSTRUCTIONS: Use a #2 pencil and completely darken the circle containing your answer choice for each question. Erase completely to change.

	A	B	C	D
1.	Ⓐ	Ⓑ	Ⓒ	Ⓓ
2.	Ⓐ	Ⓑ	Ⓒ	Ⓓ
3.	Ⓐ	Ⓑ	Ⓒ	Ⓓ
4.	Ⓐ	Ⓑ	Ⓒ	Ⓓ
5.	Ⓐ	Ⓑ	Ⓒ	Ⓓ
6.	Ⓐ	Ⓑ	Ⓒ	Ⓓ
7.	Ⓐ	Ⓑ	Ⓒ	Ⓓ
8.	Ⓐ	Ⓑ	Ⓒ	Ⓓ
9.	Ⓐ	Ⓑ	Ⓒ	Ⓓ
10.	Ⓐ	Ⓑ	Ⓒ	Ⓓ
11.	Ⓐ	Ⓑ	Ⓒ	Ⓓ
12.	Ⓐ	Ⓑ	Ⓒ	Ⓓ
13.	Ⓐ	Ⓑ	Ⓒ	Ⓓ
14.	Ⓐ	Ⓑ	Ⓒ	Ⓓ
15.	Ⓐ	Ⓑ	Ⓒ	Ⓓ
16.	Ⓐ	Ⓑ	Ⓒ	Ⓓ
17.	Ⓐ	Ⓑ	Ⓒ	Ⓓ
18.	Ⓐ	Ⓑ	Ⓒ	Ⓓ
19.	Ⓐ	Ⓑ	Ⓒ	Ⓓ
20.	Ⓐ	Ⓑ	Ⓒ	Ⓓ

Practice Exam II

Date _____

MRA Answer Sheet
Chapter 7
Classification Systems

INSTRUCTIONS: Use a #2 pencil and completely darken the circle containing your answer choice for each question. Erase completely to change.

1. Ⓐ Ⓑ Ⓒ Ⓓ
2. Ⓐ Ⓑ Ⓒ Ⓓ
3. Ⓐ Ⓑ Ⓒ Ⓓ
4. Ⓐ Ⓑ Ⓒ Ⓓ
5. Ⓐ Ⓑ Ⓒ Ⓓ
6. Ⓐ Ⓑ Ⓒ Ⓓ
7. Ⓐ Ⓑ Ⓒ Ⓓ
8. Ⓐ Ⓑ Ⓒ Ⓓ
9. Ⓐ Ⓑ Ⓒ Ⓓ
10. Ⓐ Ⓑ Ⓒ Ⓓ
11. Ⓐ Ⓑ Ⓒ Ⓓ
12. Ⓐ Ⓑ Ⓒ Ⓓ
13. Ⓐ Ⓑ Ⓒ Ⓓ
14. Ⓐ Ⓑ Ⓒ Ⓓ
15. Ⓐ Ⓑ Ⓒ Ⓓ
16. Ⓐ Ⓑ Ⓒ Ⓓ
17. Ⓐ Ⓑ Ⓒ Ⓓ
18. Ⓐ Ⓑ Ⓒ Ⓓ
19. Ⓐ Ⓑ Ⓒ Ⓓ
20. Ⓐ Ⓑ Ⓒ Ⓓ

Practice Exam II

Date _____

MRT Answer Sheet
Chapter 7
Classification Systems

INSTRUCTIONS: Use a #2 pencil and completely darken the circle containing your answer choice for each question. Erase completely to change.

1. Ⓐ Ⓑ Ⓒ Ⓓ
2. Ⓐ Ⓑ Ⓒ Ⓓ
3. Ⓐ Ⓑ Ⓒ Ⓓ
4. Ⓐ Ⓑ Ⓒ Ⓓ
5. Ⓐ Ⓑ Ⓒ Ⓓ
6. Ⓐ Ⓑ Ⓒ Ⓓ
7. Ⓐ Ⓑ Ⓒ Ⓓ
8. Ⓐ Ⓑ Ⓒ Ⓓ
9. Ⓐ Ⓑ Ⓒ Ⓓ
10. Ⓐ Ⓑ Ⓒ Ⓓ
11. Ⓐ Ⓑ Ⓒ Ⓓ
12. Ⓐ Ⓑ Ⓒ Ⓓ
13. Ⓐ Ⓑ Ⓒ Ⓓ
14. Ⓐ Ⓑ Ⓒ Ⓓ
15. Ⓐ Ⓑ Ⓒ Ⓓ
16. Ⓐ Ⓑ Ⓒ Ⓓ
17. Ⓐ Ⓑ Ⓒ Ⓓ
18. Ⓐ Ⓑ Ⓒ Ⓓ
19. Ⓐ Ⓑ Ⓒ Ⓓ
20. Ⓐ Ⓑ Ⓒ Ⓓ

Practice Exam II

Date _____

MRA Answer Sheet
Chapter 8
Coding

INSTRUCTIONS: Use a #2 pencil and completely darken the circle containing your answer choice for each question. Erase completely to change.

#	A	B	C	D		#	A	B	C	D
1.	Ⓐ	Ⓑ	Ⓒ	Ⓓ		16.	Ⓐ	Ⓑ	Ⓒ	Ⓓ
2.	Ⓐ	Ⓑ	Ⓒ	Ⓓ		17.	Ⓐ	Ⓑ	Ⓒ	Ⓓ
3.	Ⓐ	Ⓑ	Ⓒ	Ⓓ		18.	Ⓐ	Ⓑ	Ⓒ	Ⓓ
4.	Ⓐ	Ⓑ	Ⓒ	Ⓓ		19.	Ⓐ	Ⓑ	Ⓒ	Ⓓ
5.	Ⓐ	Ⓑ	Ⓒ	Ⓓ		20.	Ⓐ	Ⓑ	Ⓒ	Ⓓ
6.	Ⓐ	Ⓑ	Ⓒ	Ⓓ		21.	Ⓐ	Ⓑ	Ⓒ	Ⓓ
7.	Ⓐ	Ⓑ	Ⓒ	Ⓓ		22.	Ⓐ	Ⓑ	Ⓒ	Ⓓ
8.	Ⓐ	Ⓑ	Ⓒ	Ⓓ		23.	Ⓐ	Ⓑ	Ⓒ	Ⓓ
9.	Ⓐ	Ⓑ	Ⓒ	Ⓓ		24.	Ⓐ	Ⓑ	Ⓒ	Ⓓ
10.	Ⓐ	Ⓑ	Ⓒ	Ⓓ		25.	Ⓐ	Ⓑ	Ⓒ	Ⓓ
11.	Ⓐ	Ⓑ	Ⓒ	Ⓓ		26.	Ⓐ	Ⓑ	Ⓒ	Ⓓ
12.	Ⓐ	Ⓑ	Ⓒ	Ⓓ		27.	Ⓐ	Ⓑ	Ⓒ	Ⓓ
13.	Ⓐ	Ⓑ	Ⓒ	Ⓓ		28.	Ⓐ	Ⓑ	Ⓒ	Ⓓ
14.	Ⓐ	Ⓑ	Ⓒ	Ⓓ		29.	Ⓐ	Ⓑ	Ⓒ	Ⓓ
15.	Ⓐ	Ⓑ	Ⓒ	Ⓓ		30.	Ⓐ	Ⓑ	Ⓒ	Ⓓ

Practice Exam II

Date _____

MRT Answer Sheet
Chapter 8
Coding

INSTRUCTIONS: Use a #2 pencil and completely darken the circle containing your answer choice for each question. Erase completely to change.

#	A	B	C	D		#	A	B	C	D
1.	Ⓐ	Ⓑ	Ⓒ	Ⓓ		16.	Ⓐ	Ⓑ	Ⓒ	Ⓓ
2.	Ⓐ	Ⓑ	Ⓒ	Ⓓ		17.	Ⓐ	Ⓑ	Ⓒ	Ⓓ
3.	Ⓐ	Ⓑ	Ⓒ	Ⓓ		18.	Ⓐ	Ⓑ	Ⓒ	Ⓓ
4.	Ⓐ	Ⓑ	Ⓒ	Ⓓ		19.	Ⓐ	Ⓑ	Ⓒ	Ⓓ
5.	Ⓐ	Ⓑ	Ⓒ	Ⓓ		20.	Ⓐ	Ⓑ	Ⓒ	Ⓓ
6.	Ⓐ	Ⓑ	Ⓒ	Ⓓ		21.	Ⓐ	Ⓑ	Ⓒ	Ⓓ
7.	Ⓐ	Ⓑ	Ⓒ	Ⓓ		22.	Ⓐ	Ⓑ	Ⓒ	Ⓓ
8.	Ⓐ	Ⓑ	Ⓒ	Ⓓ		23.	Ⓐ	Ⓑ	Ⓒ	Ⓓ
9.	Ⓐ	Ⓑ	Ⓒ	Ⓓ		24.	Ⓐ	Ⓑ	Ⓒ	Ⓓ
10.	Ⓐ	Ⓑ	Ⓒ	Ⓓ		25.	Ⓐ	Ⓑ	Ⓒ	Ⓓ
11.	Ⓐ	Ⓑ	Ⓒ	Ⓓ		26.	Ⓐ	Ⓑ	Ⓒ	Ⓓ
12.	Ⓐ	Ⓑ	Ⓒ	Ⓓ		27.	Ⓐ	Ⓑ	Ⓒ	Ⓓ
13.	Ⓐ	Ⓑ	Ⓒ	Ⓓ		28.	Ⓐ	Ⓑ	Ⓒ	Ⓓ
14.	Ⓐ	Ⓑ	Ⓒ	Ⓓ		29.	Ⓐ	Ⓑ	Ⓒ	Ⓓ
15.	Ⓐ	Ⓑ	Ⓒ	Ⓓ		30.	Ⓐ	Ⓑ	Ⓒ	Ⓓ

Practice Exam II

Date _____

MRA Answer Sheet
Chapter 9
Legal Issues

INSTRUCTIONS: Use a #2 pencil and completely darken the circle containing your answer choice for each question. Erase completely to change.

1. Ⓐ Ⓑ Ⓒ Ⓓ
2. Ⓐ Ⓑ Ⓒ Ⓓ
3. Ⓐ Ⓑ Ⓒ Ⓓ
4. Ⓐ Ⓑ Ⓒ Ⓓ
5. Ⓐ Ⓑ Ⓒ Ⓓ
6. Ⓐ Ⓑ Ⓒ Ⓓ
7. Ⓐ Ⓑ Ⓒ Ⓓ
8. Ⓐ Ⓑ Ⓒ Ⓓ
9. Ⓐ Ⓑ Ⓒ Ⓓ
10. Ⓐ Ⓑ Ⓒ Ⓓ
11. Ⓐ Ⓑ Ⓒ Ⓓ
12. Ⓐ Ⓑ Ⓒ Ⓓ
13. Ⓐ Ⓑ Ⓒ Ⓓ
14. Ⓐ Ⓑ Ⓒ Ⓓ
15. Ⓐ Ⓑ Ⓒ Ⓓ
16. Ⓐ Ⓑ Ⓒ Ⓓ
17. Ⓐ Ⓑ Ⓒ Ⓓ
18. Ⓐ Ⓑ Ⓒ Ⓓ
19. Ⓐ Ⓑ Ⓒ Ⓓ
20. Ⓐ Ⓑ Ⓒ Ⓓ

Practice Exam II

Date _____

MRT Answer Sheet
Chapter 9
Legal Issues

INSTRUCTIONS: Use a #2 pencil and completely darken the circle containing your answer choice for each question. Erase completely to change.

1. Ⓐ Ⓑ Ⓒ Ⓓ
2. Ⓐ Ⓑ Ⓒ Ⓓ
3. Ⓐ Ⓑ Ⓒ Ⓓ
4. Ⓐ Ⓑ Ⓒ Ⓓ
5. Ⓐ Ⓑ Ⓒ Ⓓ
6. Ⓐ Ⓑ Ⓒ Ⓓ
7. Ⓐ Ⓑ Ⓒ Ⓓ
8. Ⓐ Ⓑ Ⓒ Ⓓ
9. Ⓐ Ⓑ Ⓒ Ⓓ
10. Ⓐ Ⓑ Ⓒ Ⓓ
11. Ⓐ Ⓑ Ⓒ Ⓓ
12. Ⓐ Ⓑ Ⓒ Ⓓ
13. Ⓐ Ⓑ Ⓒ Ⓓ
14. Ⓐ Ⓑ Ⓒ Ⓓ
15. Ⓐ Ⓑ Ⓒ Ⓓ
16. Ⓐ Ⓑ Ⓒ Ⓓ
17. Ⓐ Ⓑ Ⓒ Ⓓ
18. Ⓐ Ⓑ Ⓒ Ⓓ
19. Ⓐ Ⓑ Ⓒ Ⓓ
20. Ⓐ Ⓑ Ⓒ Ⓓ

Practice Exam II

Date _____

MRA Answer Sheet
Chapter 10
Management

INSTRUCTIONS: Use a #2 pencil and completely darken the circle containing your answer choice for each question. Erase completely to change.

#	A	B	C	D		#	A	B	C	D
1.	Ⓐ	Ⓑ	Ⓒ	Ⓓ		16.	Ⓐ	Ⓑ	Ⓒ	Ⓓ
2.	Ⓐ	Ⓑ	Ⓒ	Ⓓ		17.	Ⓐ	Ⓑ	Ⓒ	Ⓓ
3.	Ⓐ	Ⓑ	Ⓒ	Ⓓ		18.	Ⓐ	Ⓑ	Ⓒ	Ⓓ
4.	Ⓐ	Ⓑ	Ⓒ	Ⓓ		19.	Ⓐ	Ⓑ	Ⓒ	Ⓓ
5.	Ⓐ	Ⓑ	Ⓒ	Ⓓ		20.	Ⓐ	Ⓑ	Ⓒ	Ⓓ
6.	Ⓐ	Ⓑ	Ⓒ	Ⓓ		21.	Ⓐ	Ⓑ	Ⓒ	Ⓓ
7.	Ⓐ	Ⓑ	Ⓒ	Ⓓ		22.	Ⓐ	Ⓑ	Ⓒ	Ⓓ
8.	Ⓐ	Ⓑ	Ⓒ	Ⓓ		23.	Ⓐ	Ⓑ	Ⓒ	Ⓓ
9.	Ⓐ	Ⓑ	Ⓒ	Ⓓ		24.	Ⓐ	Ⓑ	Ⓒ	Ⓓ
10.	Ⓐ	Ⓑ	Ⓒ	Ⓓ		25.	Ⓐ	Ⓑ	Ⓒ	Ⓓ
11.	Ⓐ	Ⓑ	Ⓒ	Ⓓ
12.	Ⓐ	Ⓑ	Ⓒ	Ⓓ
13.	Ⓐ	Ⓑ	Ⓒ	Ⓓ
14.	Ⓐ	Ⓑ	Ⓒ	Ⓓ
15.	Ⓐ	Ⓑ	Ⓒ	Ⓓ

Practice Exam II

Date _____

MRT Answer Sheet
Chapter 10
Management

INSTRUCTIONS: Use a #2 pencil and completely darken the circle containing your answer choice for each question. Erase completely to change.

#	A	B	C	D		#	A	B	C	D
1.	Ⓐ	Ⓑ	Ⓒ	Ⓓ		16.	Ⓐ	Ⓑ	Ⓒ	Ⓓ
2.	Ⓐ	Ⓑ	Ⓒ	Ⓓ		17.	Ⓐ	Ⓑ	Ⓒ	Ⓓ
3.	Ⓐ	Ⓑ	Ⓒ	Ⓓ		18.	Ⓐ	Ⓑ	Ⓒ	Ⓓ
4.	Ⓐ	Ⓑ	Ⓒ	Ⓓ		19.	Ⓐ	Ⓑ	Ⓒ	Ⓓ
5.	Ⓐ	Ⓑ	Ⓒ	Ⓓ		20.	Ⓐ	Ⓑ	Ⓒ	Ⓓ
6.	Ⓐ	Ⓑ	Ⓒ	Ⓓ		21.	Ⓐ	Ⓑ	Ⓒ	Ⓓ
7.	Ⓐ	Ⓑ	Ⓒ	Ⓓ		22.	Ⓐ	Ⓑ	Ⓒ	Ⓓ
8.	Ⓐ	Ⓑ	Ⓒ	Ⓓ		23.	Ⓐ	Ⓑ	Ⓒ	Ⓓ
9.	Ⓐ	Ⓑ	Ⓒ	Ⓓ		24.	Ⓐ	Ⓑ	Ⓒ	Ⓓ
10.	Ⓐ	Ⓑ	Ⓒ	Ⓓ		25.	Ⓐ	Ⓑ	Ⓒ	Ⓓ
11.	Ⓐ	Ⓑ	Ⓒ	Ⓓ						
12.	Ⓐ	Ⓑ	Ⓒ	Ⓓ						
13.	Ⓐ	Ⓑ	Ⓒ	Ⓓ						
14.	Ⓐ	Ⓑ	Ⓒ	Ⓓ						
15.	Ⓐ	Ⓑ	Ⓒ	Ⓓ						

Practice Exam II

Date _____

MRA Answer Sheet
Chapter 11
Human Resource Management

INSTRUCTIONS: Use a #2 pencil and completely darken the circle containing your answer choice for each question. Erase completely to change.

#	A	B	C	D
1.	Ⓐ	Ⓑ	Ⓒ	Ⓓ
2.	Ⓐ	Ⓑ	Ⓒ	Ⓓ
3.	Ⓐ	Ⓑ	Ⓒ	Ⓓ
4.	Ⓐ	Ⓑ	Ⓒ	Ⓓ
5.	Ⓐ	Ⓑ	Ⓒ	Ⓓ
6.	Ⓐ	Ⓑ	Ⓒ	Ⓓ
7.	Ⓐ	Ⓑ	Ⓒ	Ⓓ
8.	Ⓐ	Ⓑ	Ⓒ	Ⓓ
9.	Ⓐ	Ⓑ	Ⓒ	Ⓓ
10.	Ⓐ	Ⓑ	Ⓒ	Ⓓ
11.	Ⓐ	Ⓑ	Ⓒ	Ⓓ
12.	Ⓐ	Ⓑ	Ⓒ	Ⓓ
13.	Ⓐ	Ⓑ	Ⓒ	Ⓓ
14.	Ⓐ	Ⓑ	Ⓒ	Ⓓ
15.	Ⓐ	Ⓑ	Ⓒ	Ⓓ
16.	Ⓐ	Ⓑ	Ⓒ	Ⓓ
17.	Ⓐ	Ⓑ	Ⓒ	Ⓓ
18.	Ⓐ	Ⓑ	Ⓒ	Ⓓ
19.	Ⓐ	Ⓑ	Ⓒ	Ⓓ
20.	Ⓐ	Ⓑ	Ⓒ	Ⓓ

Practice Exam II

Date _____

MRT Answer Sheet
Chapter 11
Human Resource Management

INSTRUCTIONS: Use a #2 pencil and completely darken the circle containing your answer choice for each question. Erase completely to change.

	A	B	C	D
1.	Ⓐ	Ⓑ	Ⓒ	Ⓓ
2.	Ⓐ	Ⓑ	Ⓒ	Ⓓ
3.	Ⓐ	Ⓑ	Ⓒ	Ⓓ
4.	Ⓐ	Ⓑ	Ⓒ	Ⓓ
5.	Ⓐ	Ⓑ	Ⓒ	Ⓓ
6.	Ⓐ	Ⓑ	Ⓒ	Ⓓ
7.	Ⓐ	Ⓑ	Ⓒ	Ⓓ
8.	Ⓐ	Ⓑ	Ⓒ	Ⓓ
9.	Ⓐ	Ⓑ	Ⓒ	Ⓓ
10.	Ⓐ	Ⓑ	Ⓒ	Ⓓ
11.	Ⓐ	Ⓑ	Ⓒ	Ⓓ
12.	Ⓐ	Ⓑ	Ⓒ	Ⓓ
13.	Ⓐ	Ⓑ	Ⓒ	Ⓓ
14.	Ⓐ	Ⓑ	Ⓒ	Ⓓ
15.	Ⓐ	Ⓑ	Ⓒ	Ⓓ
16.	Ⓐ	Ⓑ	Ⓒ	Ⓓ
17.	Ⓐ	Ⓑ	Ⓒ	Ⓓ
18.	Ⓐ	Ⓑ	Ⓒ	Ⓓ
19.	Ⓐ	Ⓑ	Ⓒ	Ⓓ
20.	Ⓐ	Ⓑ	Ⓒ	Ⓓ

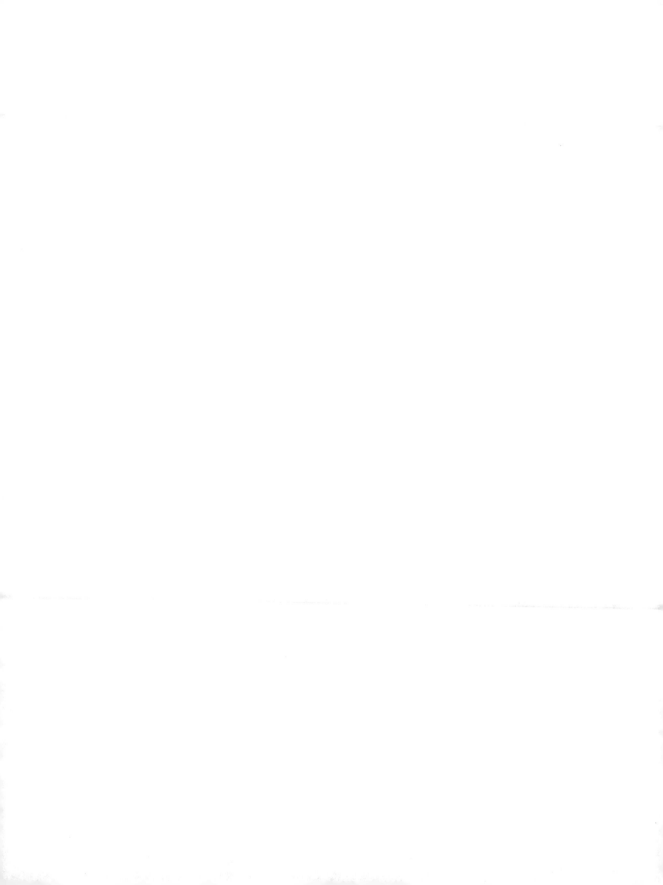